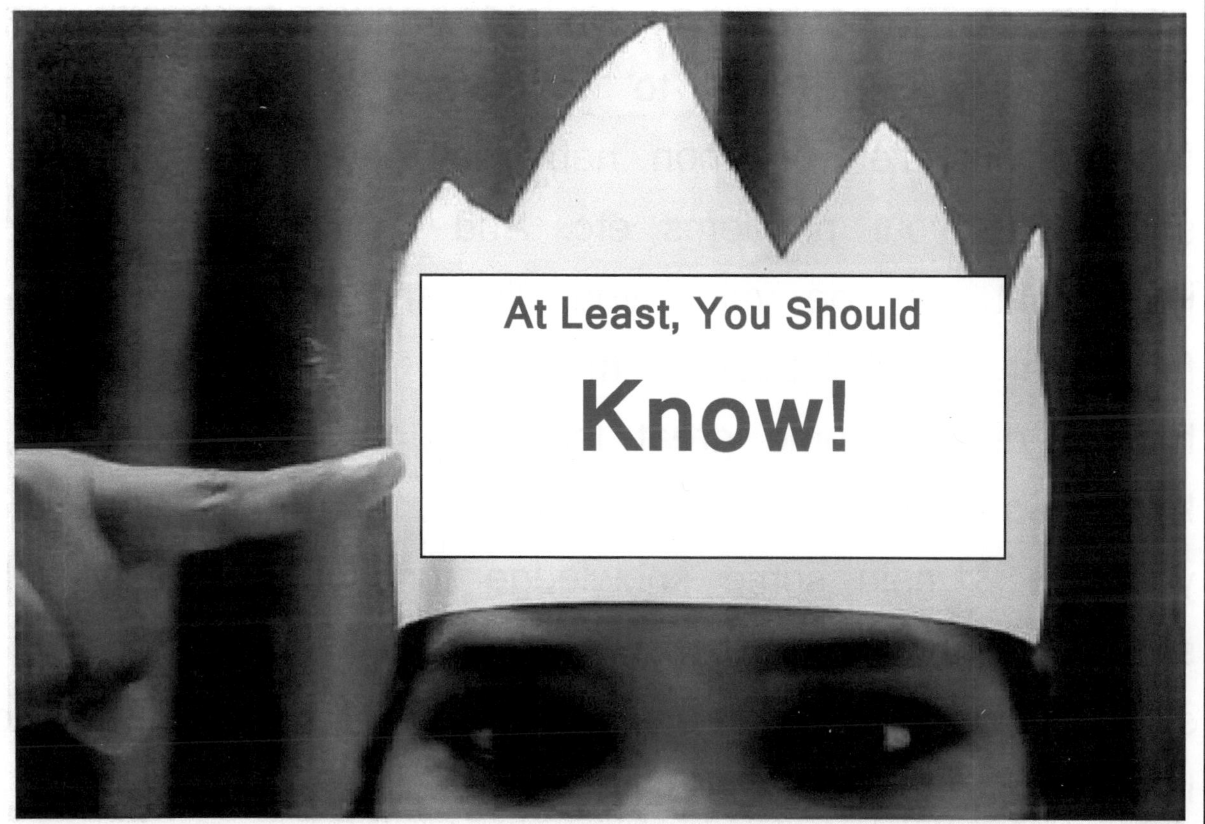

(Health Book)

Sunita Thankappan

Hello Readers, Viewers & Doers!

The book, "At Least, You Should Know!" its health book that will help you to understand the importance of food in our diet, common habits and some quick solution to your problems etc. And I am happy to know that you too value your life and want to change for better. In this book, I mentioned the common healthy diet & some great learning that we all should know. So please move forward and take best step of your life & gain some knowledge for healthy lifestyle. I shared some healthy tips with you to live your life simple, happy and for every individual in the earth who is looking for some basic healthy solution. I prepared this book based on my own knowledge, research and experience that I had with people who faced it and I had been good support to them. I can assure this book will guide & give you some right approach to live a simple & beautiful life. This small book will definitely guide you & your family to live healthy life; don't just follow but act on daily basis. Time will help you to show the results. I feel this book should keep it handy to act it.

"Connect with God if you want to live peaceful life there is no peace without him."

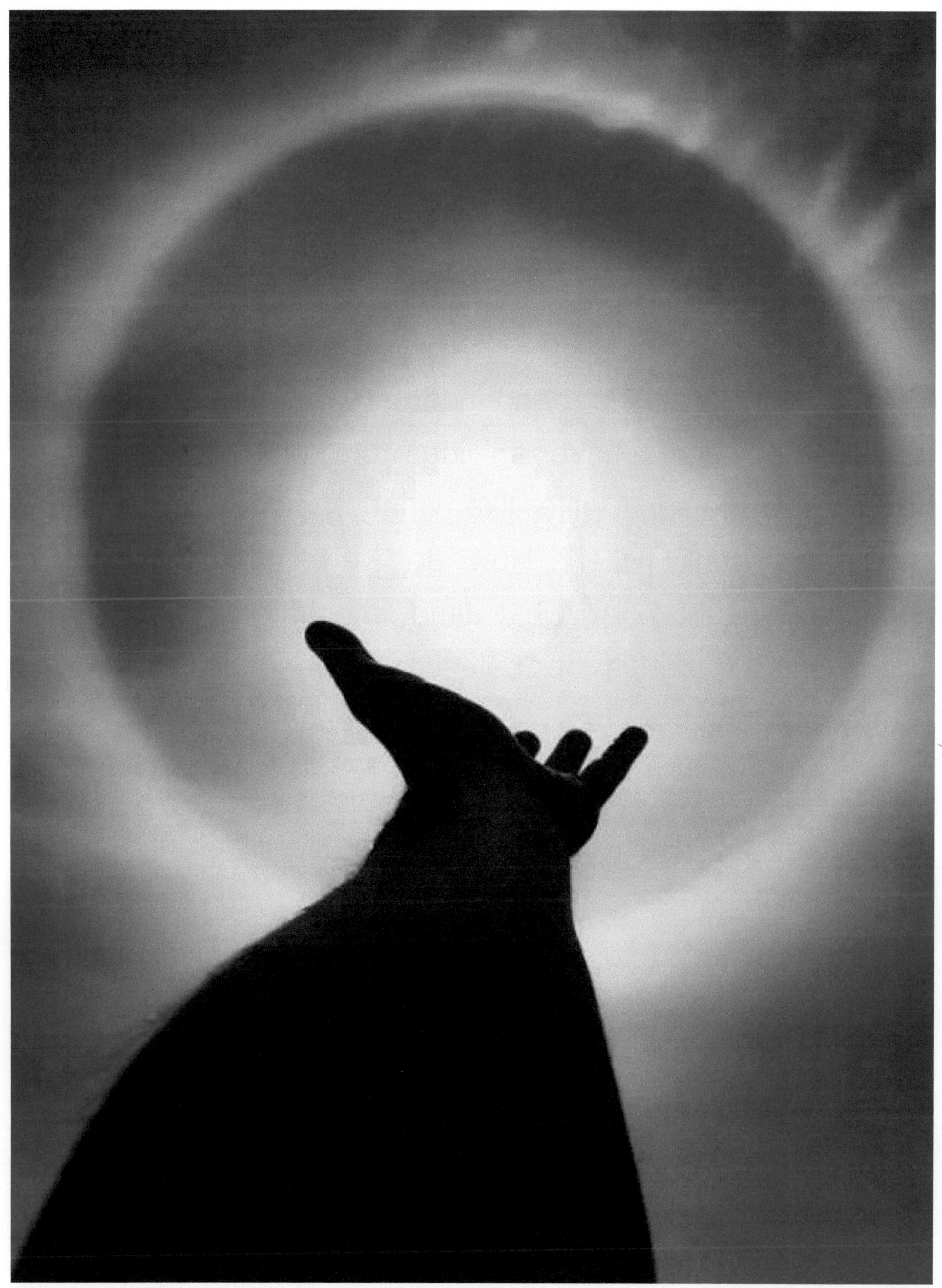

First of all, thank you for choosing this book. It's great job!

I covered the basic healthy tips to improve your health. I am not a doctor but I love to share some knowledge I gained throughout these years to treat people & myself.

Most of the mistakes happened and we did in our life because we didn't have an idea or right guidance; how do we live balanced life like what should we eat? How should we drink water? How do we control our negative thoughts? At what time should we sleep? Etc. There should always be balance between our body & soul; fresh food & fresh positive thoughts.

So what do you think, if we get the right guidance at right time, our lifestyle would be totally different, isn't it?

Yes, of course.

So I will try to guide you with some helpful & healthy tips to make your life simple & happy.

Let's get started.........

First rule of life.... Believe in God

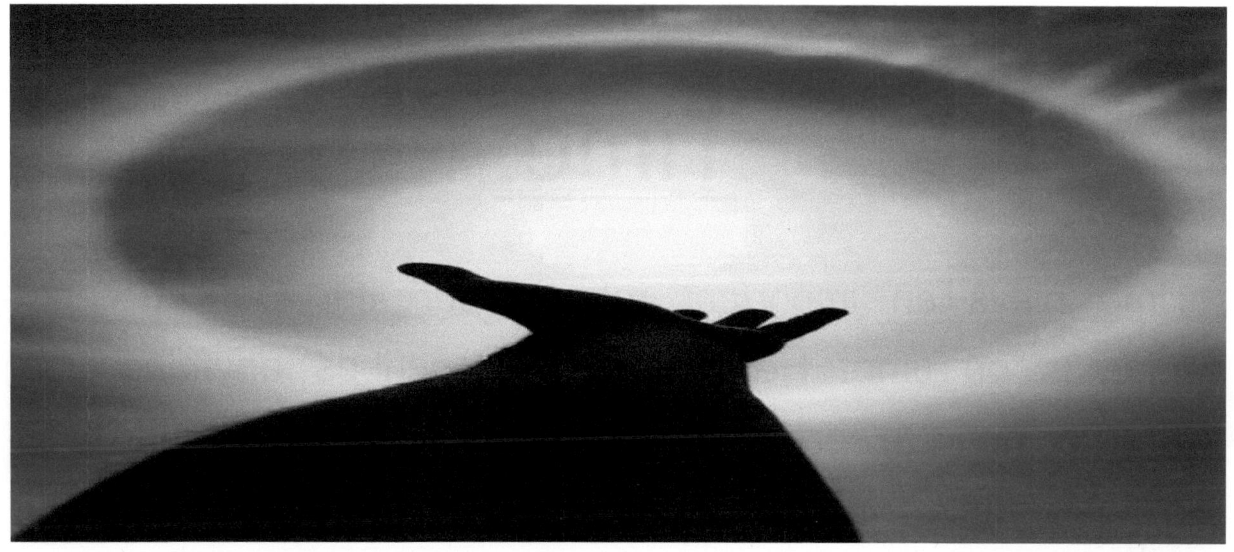

Next, to live happy in this world......

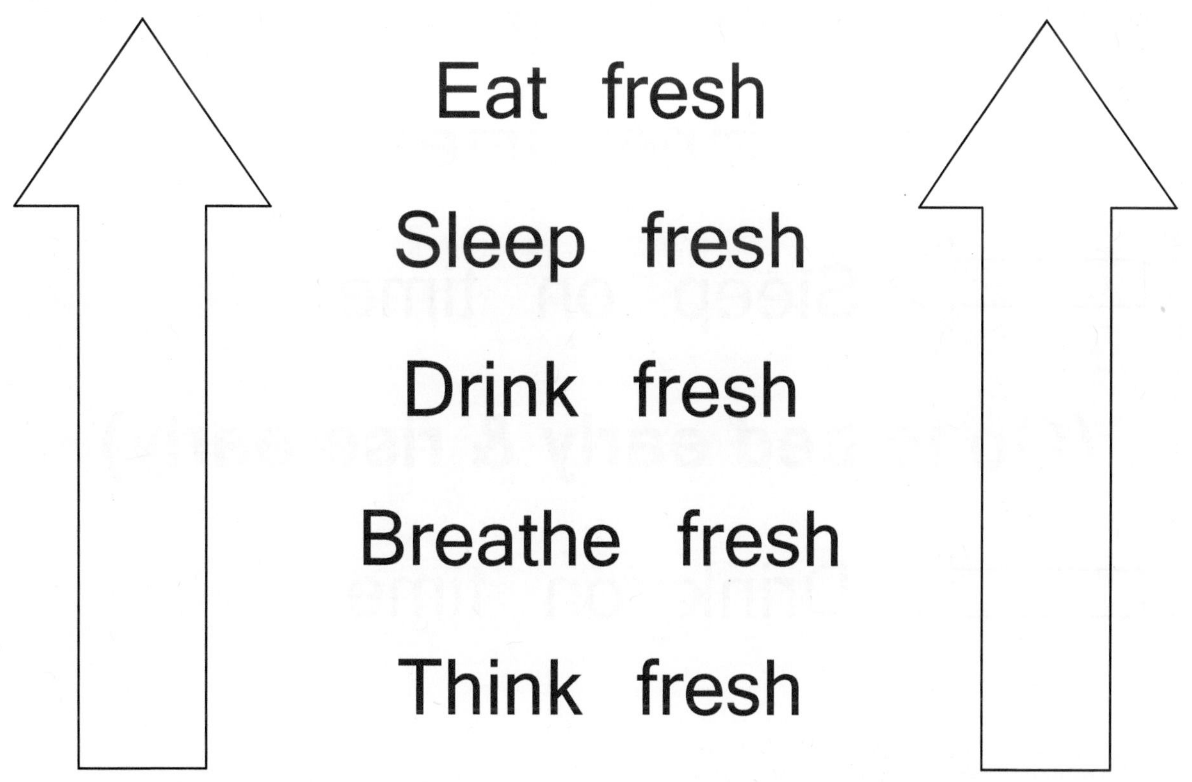

Next, schedule your time for whatever you do; value your time & of others.

Time:

Time plays an important role in our life. Our success depends on time. Here success describes anything you want to achieve emotionally, socially, physically on time. So learn time management, it is important factor in our life, so schedule your time to do your things on time.

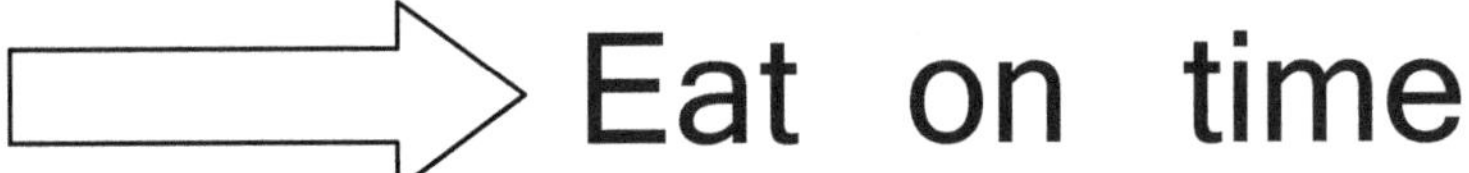

Eat on time

(Schedule your breakfast, lunch & dinner time)

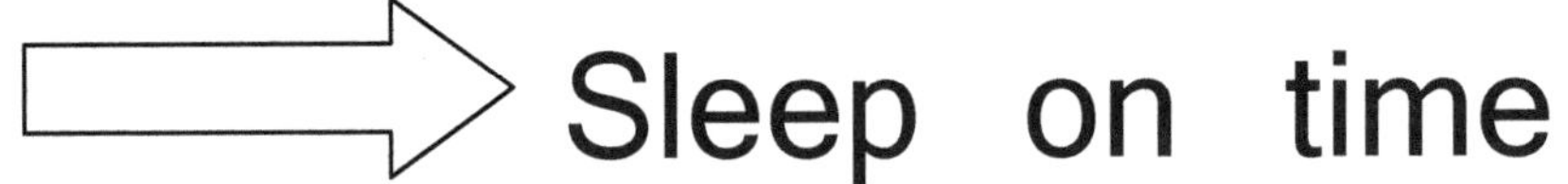

Sleep on time

(Go to bed early & rise early)

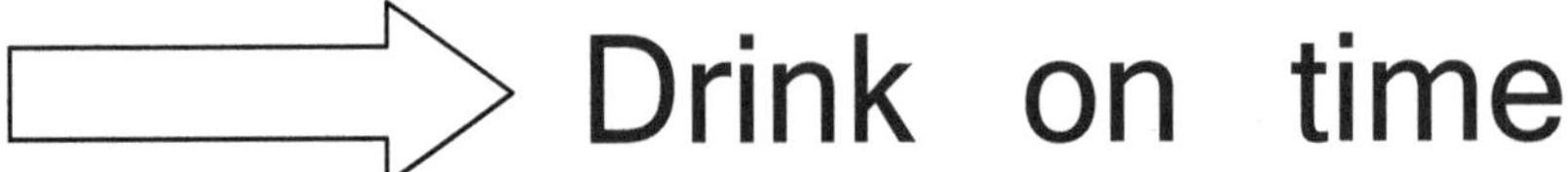

Drink on time

(Drink when you are thirsty & drink water sip by sip)

⇒ Breathe well on time

(Take some time to breathe in & breathe out in fresh air)

⇒ Think well on time

(Act well at right time)

Be peaceful most of the time.

Next, to handle every situation of life we need to learn to control our thoughts.

How to control our fast thoughts?

Does breathing exercises help us? I would say YES because it will help you to control your thoughts & relax yourself. So every day be present to feel breathe in & breathe out.

Thoughts play an important rule:

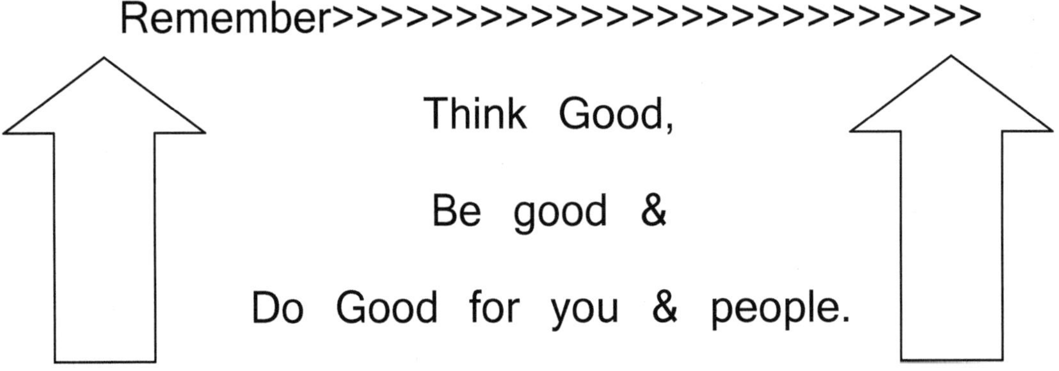

Next, hydrate yourself throughout the day.

How do we drink water?

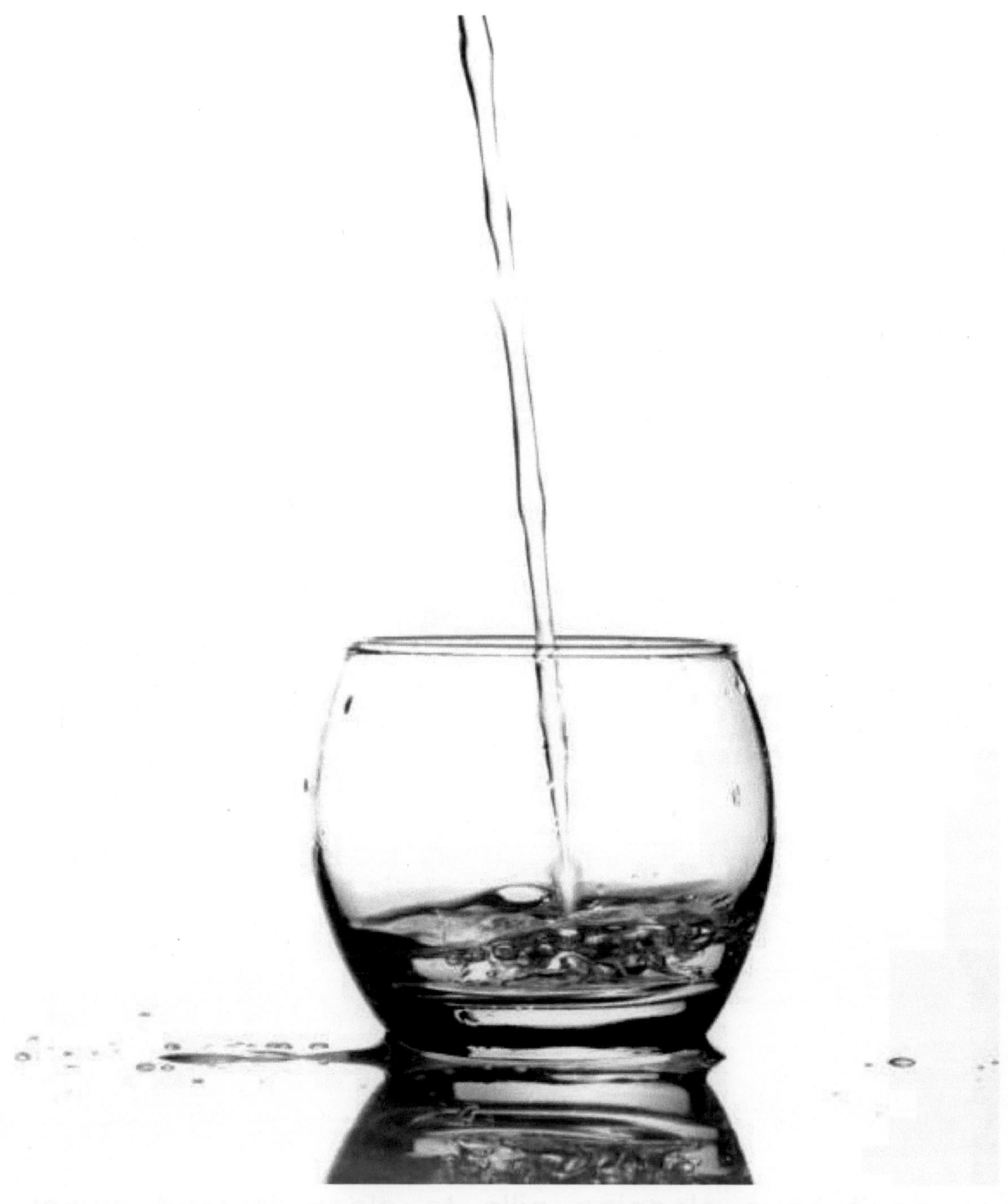

Drink water sip by sip; don't drink whole water at one shot.

Next, manage your sleep well.

How do we sleep?

Complete 8 hours of sleep help you to work best for the next day.

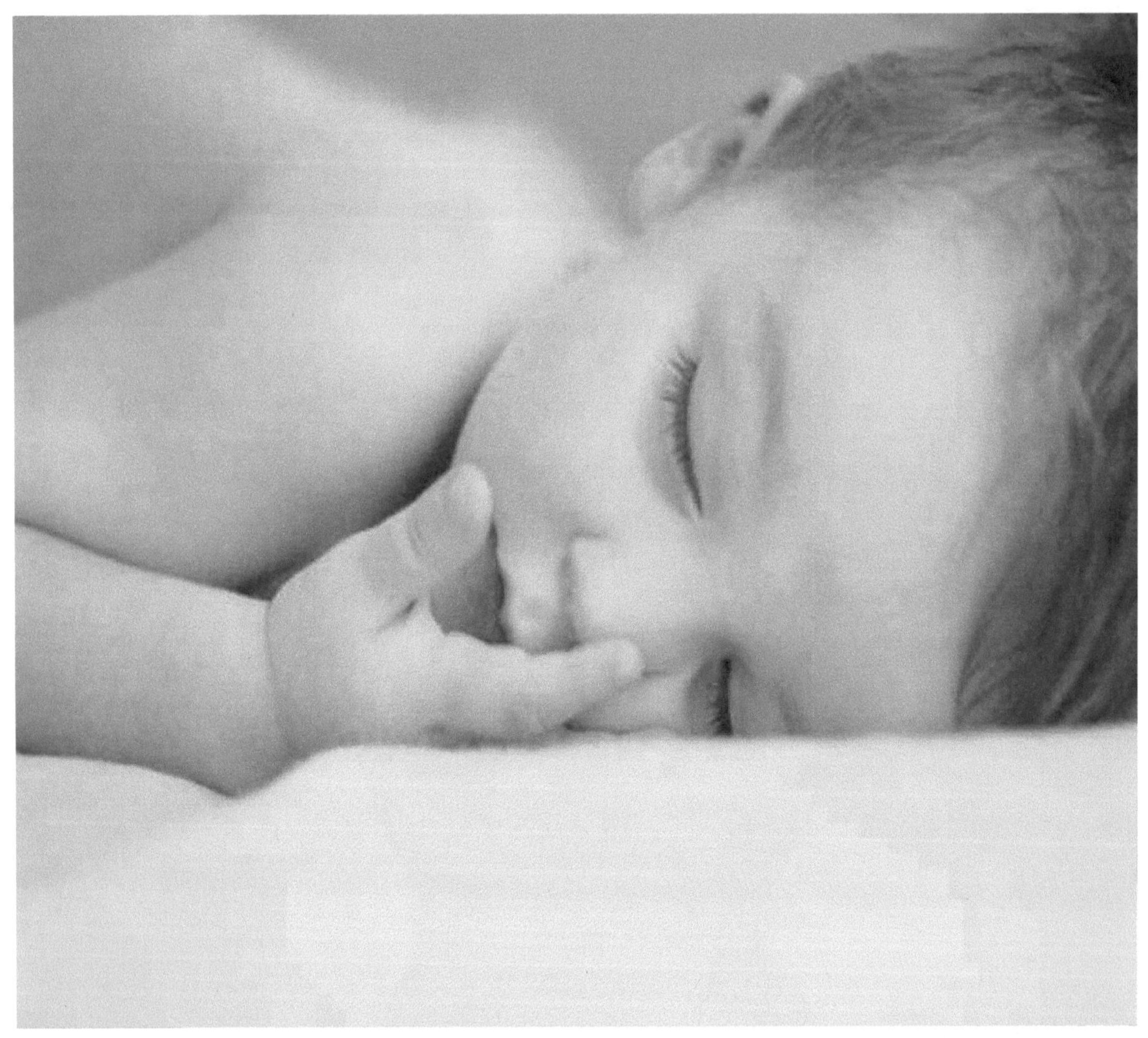

Please don't have sleeping pills to sleep instead sweat yourself/ work hard/ don't sit in one place for longer time throughout the day to have peaceful sleep.

Next, plan a well balanced diet for you, your family members.

How do we eat food?

A healthy balanced diet that includes fruits, vegetables, nuts, grains etc that help you to maintain your body in better way and can live stress free life.

Don’t overfill your stomach, keep your stomach little empty, chew your food, it will help your body to digest the food easily.

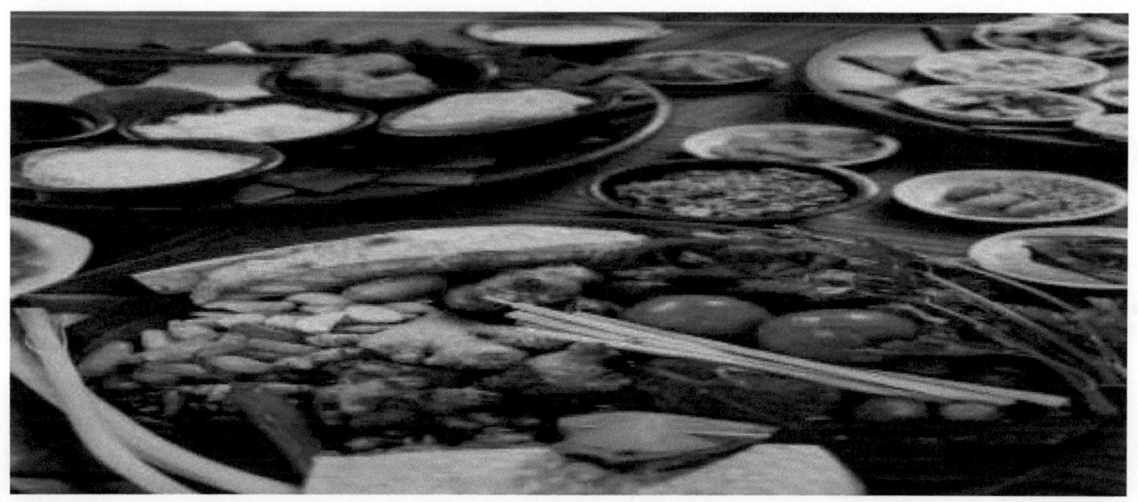

When we talk about Food, our nature has given us loads of fruits & vegetables and other essential grains, nuts, spices etc. to live wonderful life but most of the people like to eat preservatives food that leads them to live unhealthy life.

You can try some Morning, Afternoon, and Night Food to improve your health.

Best Morning food?

You can try this morning food for your better health.

Have Brown Bread sandwich & 1 fruit.

Or Idli & 1 fruit

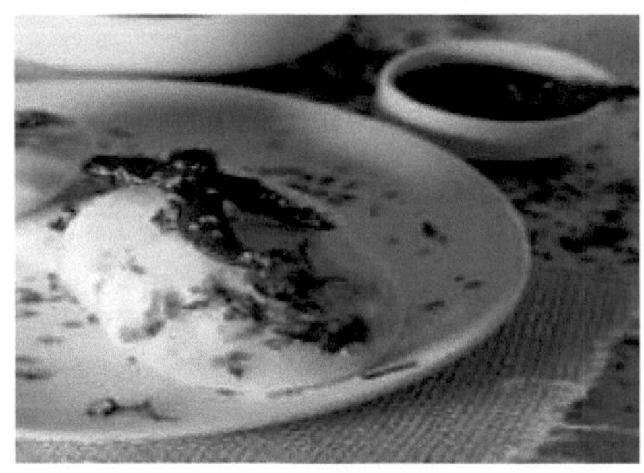

Or Chapati & vegetable, and (Any 1 seasonal Fruit of your choice)

At 12 noon you can have some seasonal fruit juice.

You can plan or write your own morning diet & follow it.

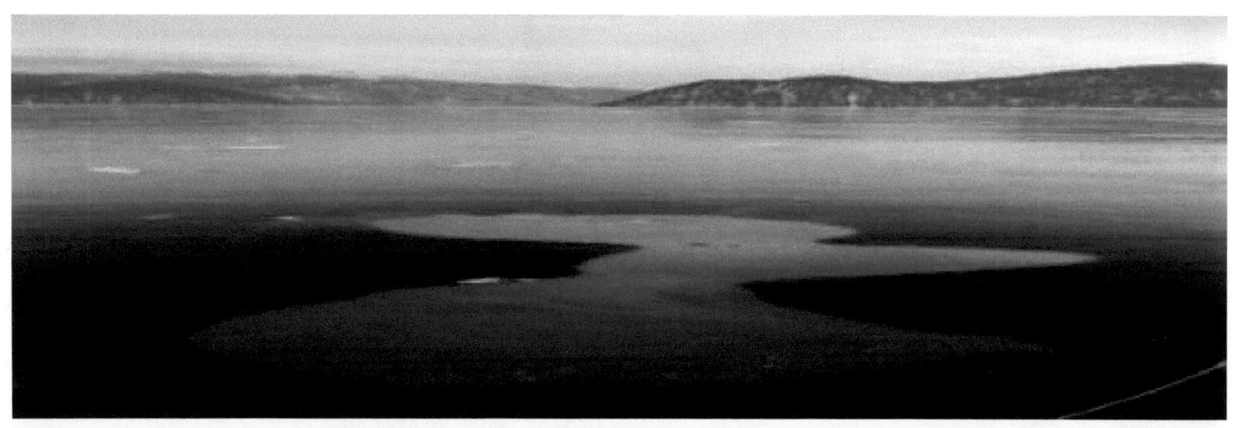

Best Afternoon Food?

You can try this plan for your diet,

Salad, Chapati, 2 varieties of Vegetables of your choice, Brown Rice, Legumes/ Pulses/ Dal, Butter milk.

In the evening, you can have some vegetables smoothie with nuts.

You can plan or write your Afternoon diet & follow it.

____

____

____

____

____

____

Or you can start with traditional food for a change....

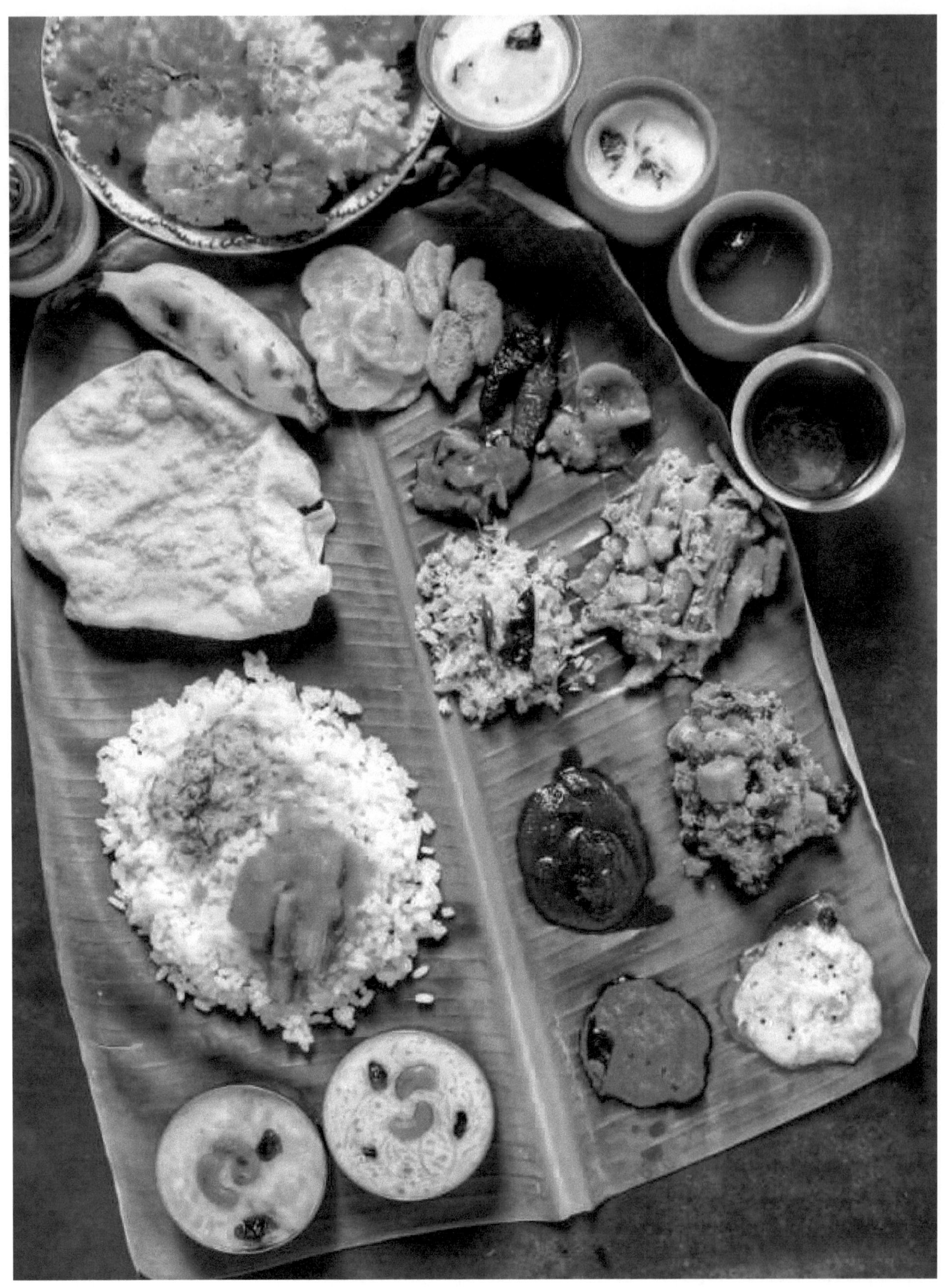

Best Night Food?

Salad or Sprouts.

These are some common diet I have added but you can try your own balanced diet but make sure avoid those things which are harmful for your body.

You can plan your Night diet & follow it.

⊗ Please Avoid These Things Completely because your body dislikes it.

1) Salt: White salt

(Use Pink & Black salt)

2) Sugar: White sugar

(Use Candy Sugar or Jaggery)

3) All Purpose Flour

(Use other grains flour)

Next, Best Exercises?

Learn Surya Namaskar

(You can check YouTube videos for Surya Namaskar)

Next, Best Yoga?

Most common I have listed i.e. Kapalabathi, Anulom Vilom, Brastika Pranayam, you can add yours.

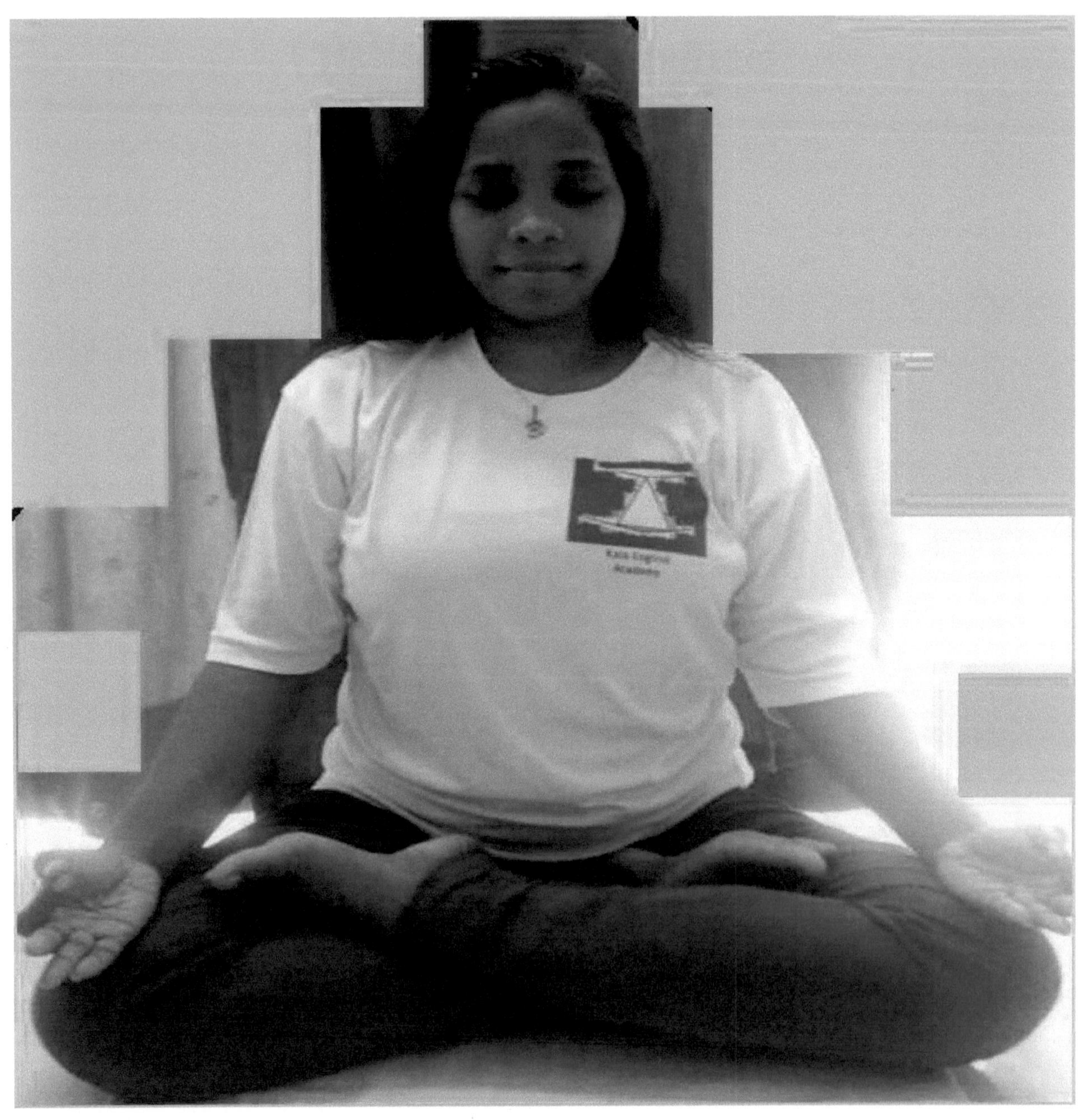

Next, Best Oil Massage?

You can do massage with Coconut oil, lemon oil, Til /Sesame oil or Mustard oil for better blood circulation.

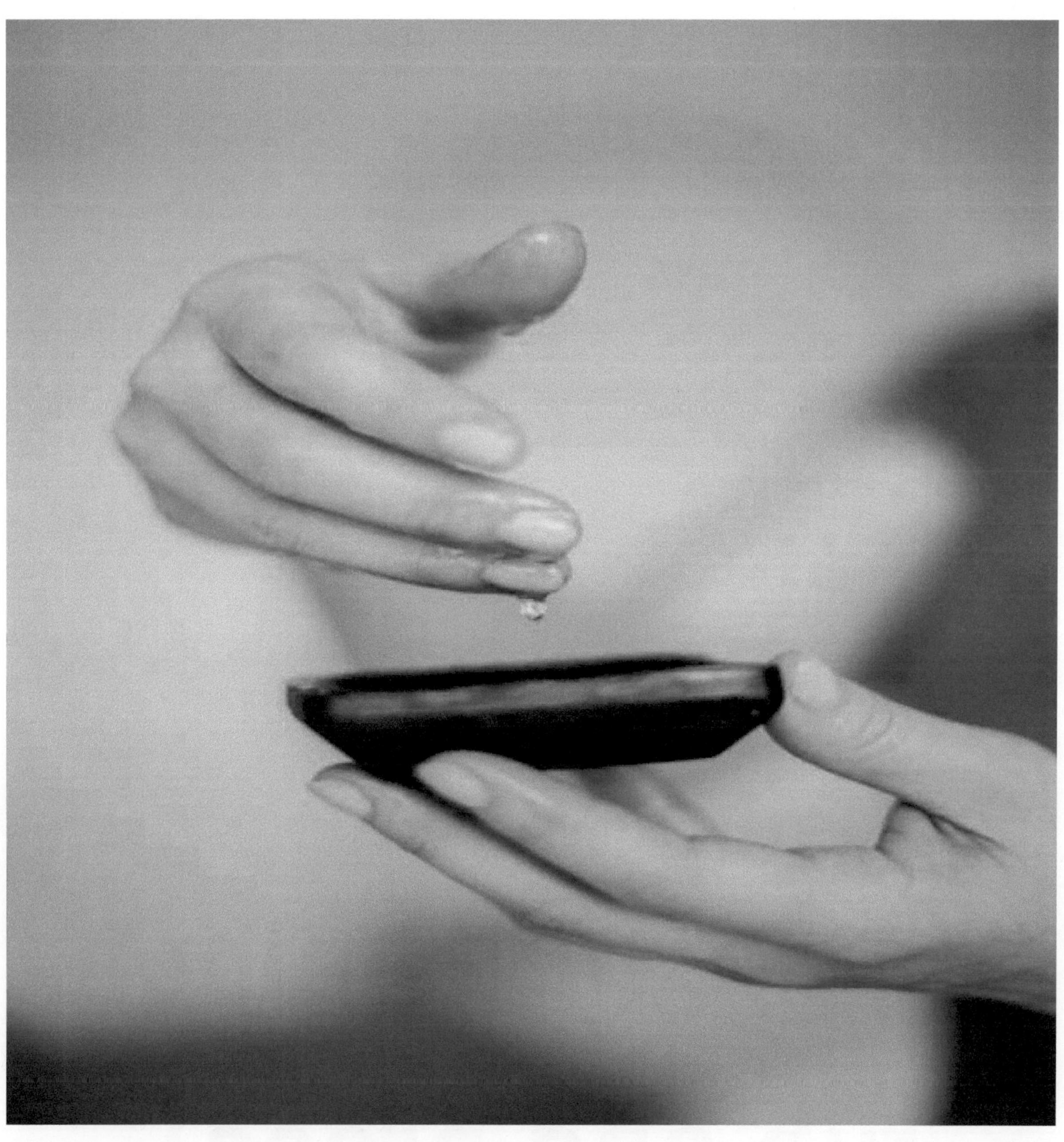

Say Hello to your Ears!!!!

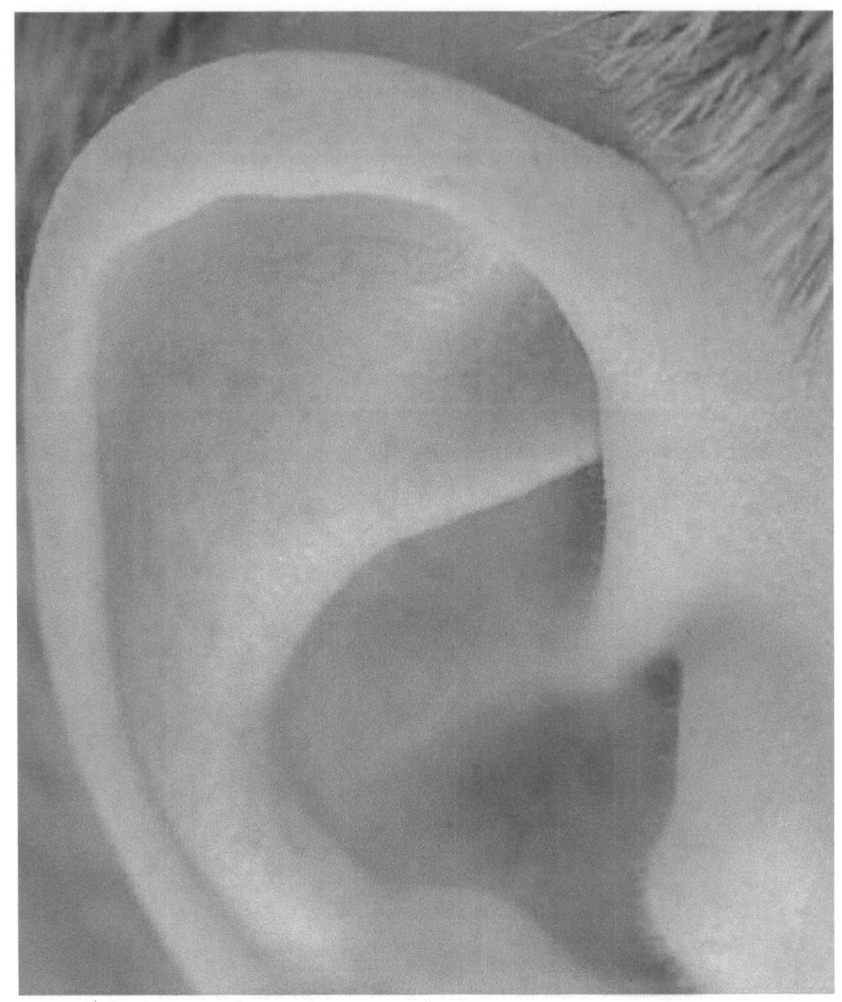

Massage your ears on daily basis, will keep you refresh, energetic & relax.

(Shake, pull, pinch, rub and press)

Next, we will now know, what are the best foods we should have for some organs.

All organs of our body is important but some of the most important organs that we mostly take care, or show concern & spend our valuable time, that I have listed below:

1) Eyes
2) Hair
3) Skin
4) Bones
5) Stomach
6) Heart
7) Muscles

Let's learn, what are the best fruits, vegetables, nuts, massage etc. for these organs....

1) Eyes

Eyes Healthy Food

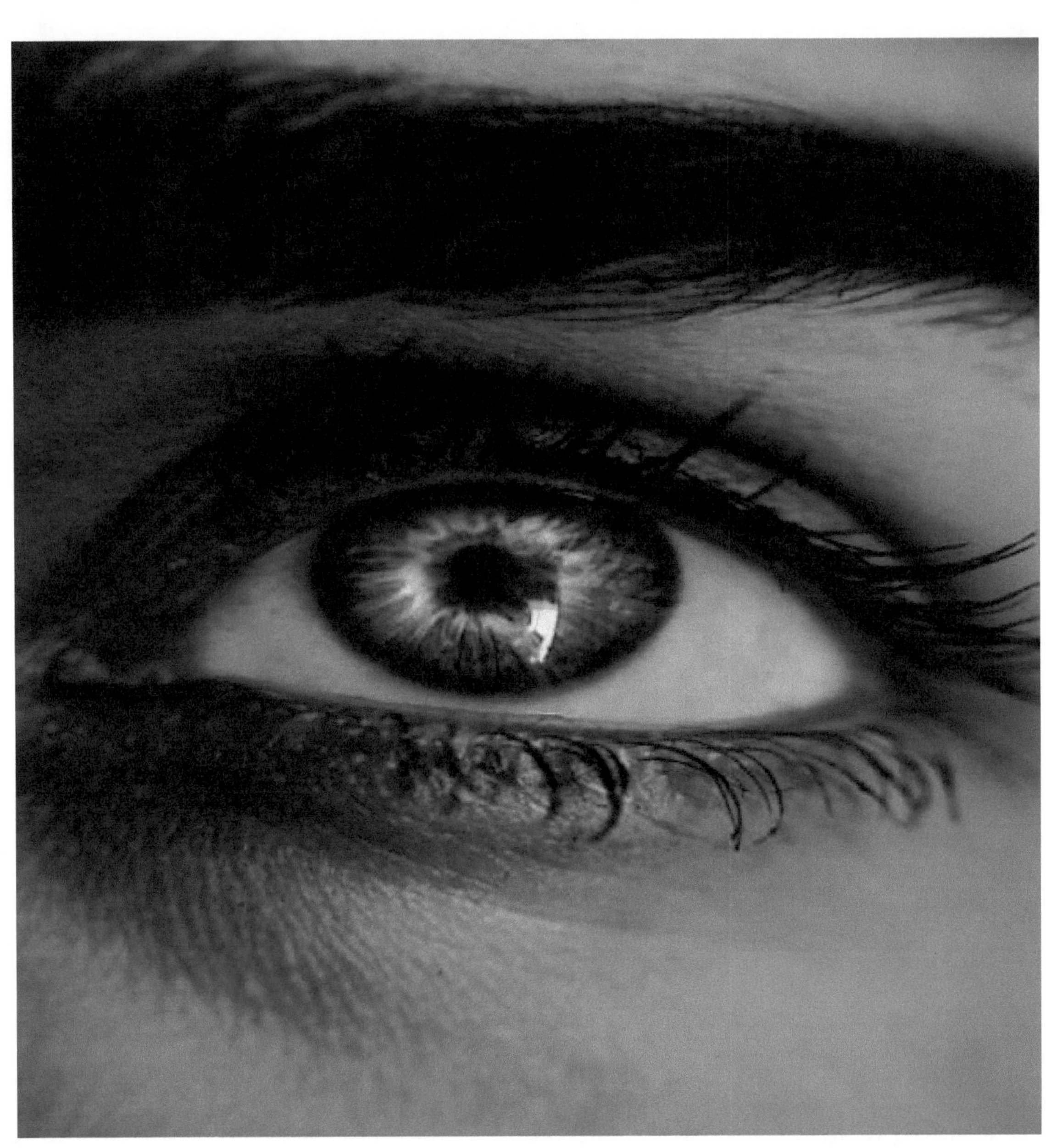

Best Fruit for eyes:

Fruits contain powerful antioxidants that help detoxify the skin; it gives fresh look and keeps it in good health.

1) Orange juice
2) Eat a banana daily
3) Apples
4) Grapes
5) Gooseberries

Best Vegetables for eyes:

The below vegetables will improve your eyesight, keep your eyes strong,

1) Spinach
2) Kale
3) Other dark green leafy vegetables
4) Carrot
5) Sweet Potato

Best nuts & seeds for eyes:

Some nuts help to improve your eyesight & prevent from cataract and eye muscle degeneration.

1) Almonds
2) Apricots
3) Cashew nuts

Best Massage for eyes:

1) Tap with your index and middle fingers, tap out a circle around your eyes.

Best Exercises for eyes:

1) Blink your eyes for 30 seconds.

2) Rub your palms for 2 minutes & keep it on your eyes

3) Roll your eyes up, down, left & right, next while sitting or standing move your eyes in a clockwise direction 5 times making the circle as wide as you can. Do it in the morning.

Acupressure Point for eyes:

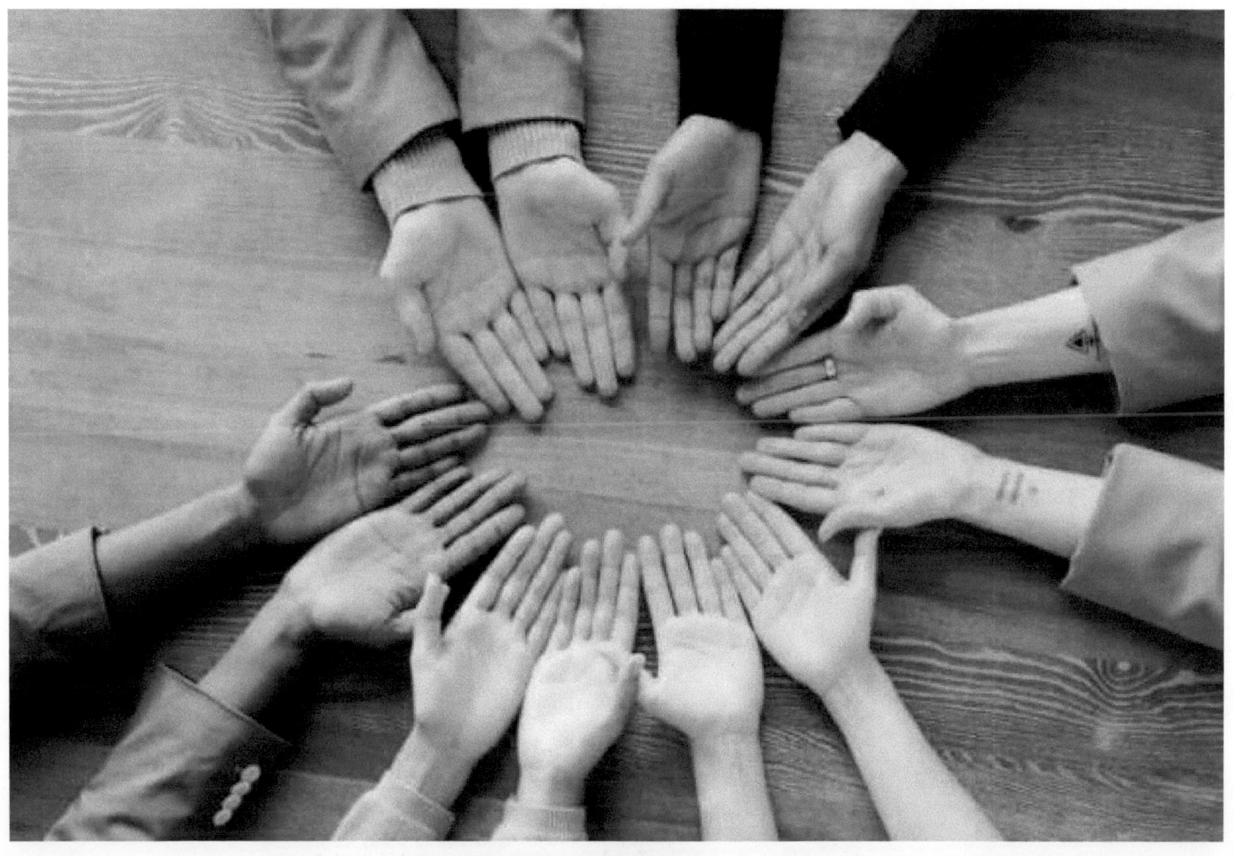

We all should try & learn acupressure that helps us to get relieve from pain in our body.

(You can watch YouTube videos for Some Common Acupressure Points of eyes) or press the star points which has shown in the pictures mentioned below.

1)

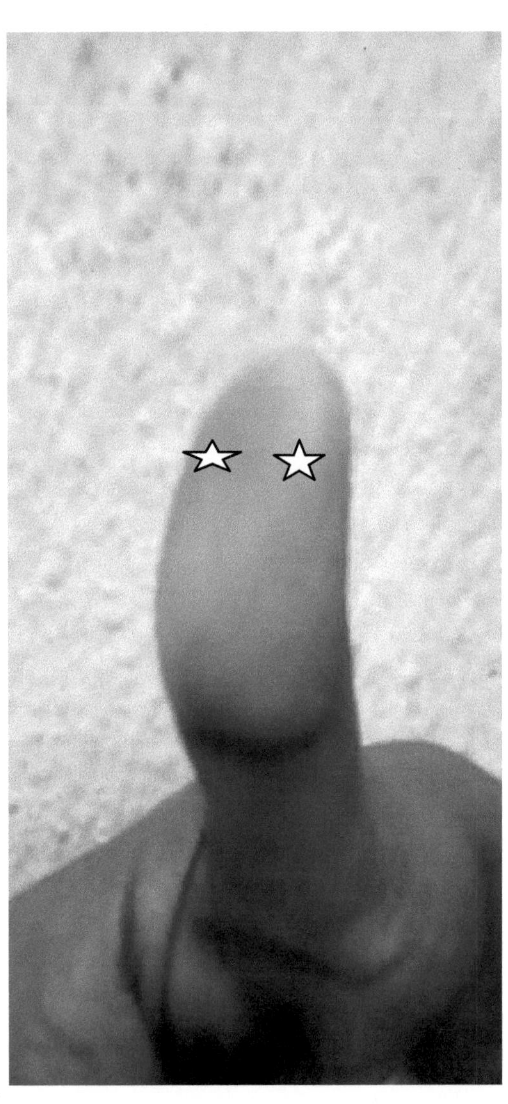

2)

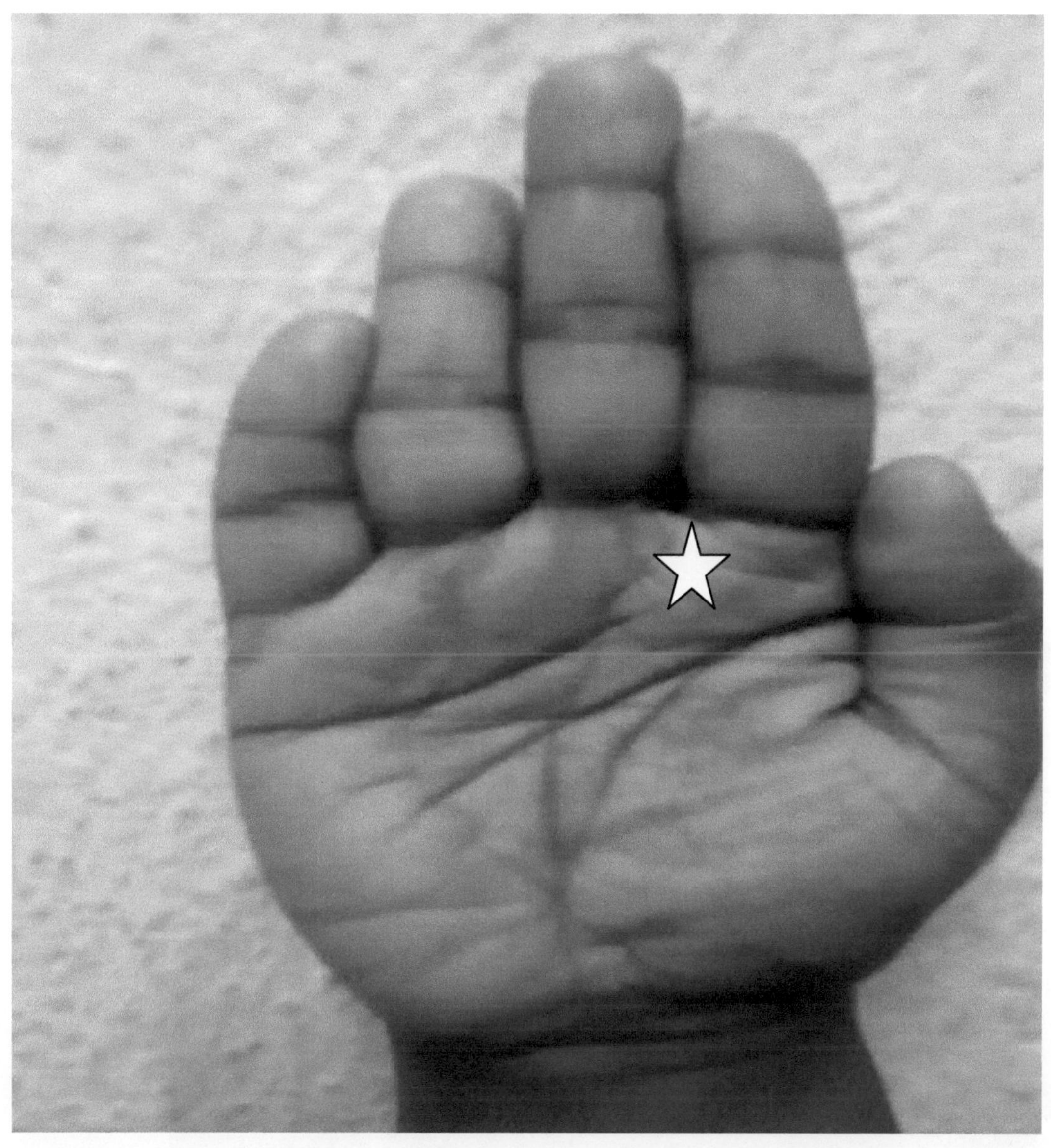

Locate these star points on your thumb & palm and stimulate these points, just press these points for 15 seconds and release, continue this process for 5 to 10 minutes on regular basis.

Affirm the Affirmation

Affirmation helps to control your negative thoughts!

Thank you God,

I am happy, healthy & have perfect vision of life.

Connect yourself with God so you will always act right at the right moment.

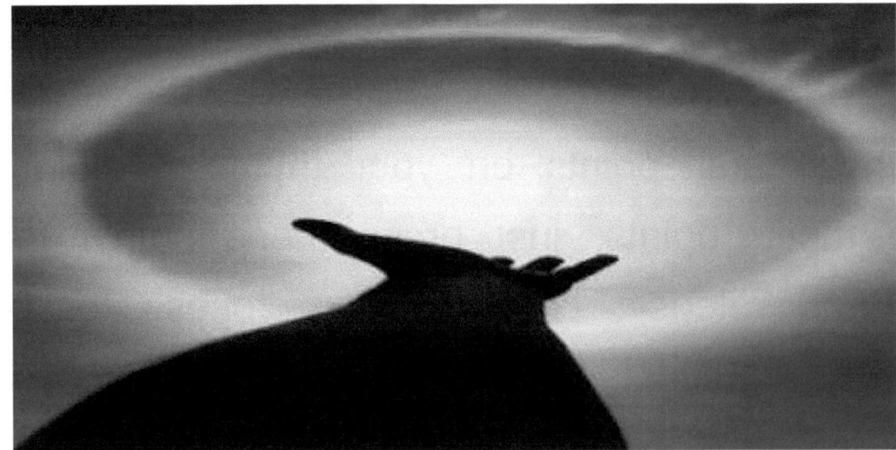

2) Hair Healthy Food

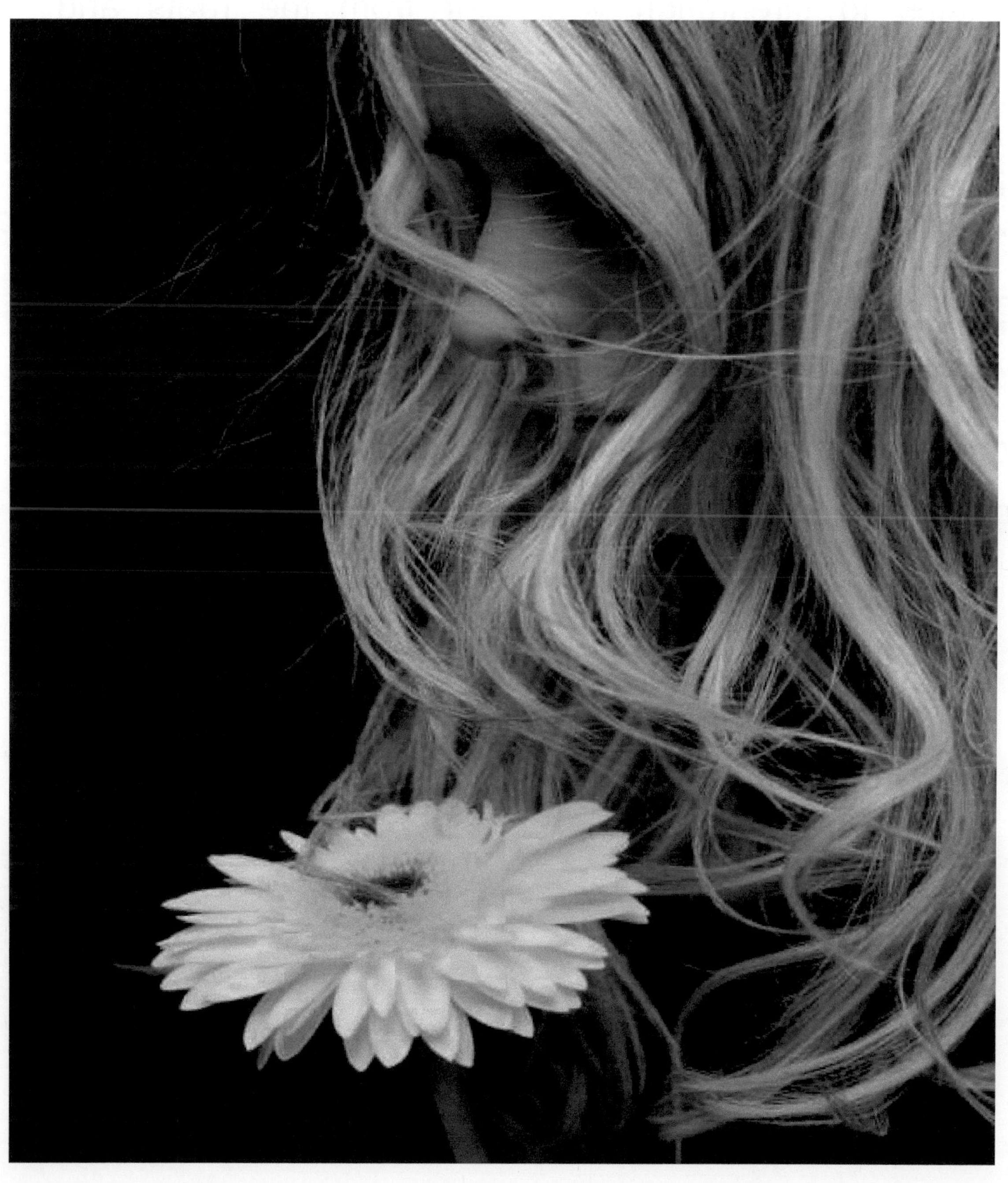

Best Fruit for your hair:

It helps to strengthen your hair from the roots and prevent from hair damage. Fruits for hair growth will improve blood circulation of our whole body.

Orange is the best fruit for hair it nourishes and grows long strong healthy hair and this fruit is easily available throughout the year.

Some other fruits that help to grow your hair faster and make your hair soft & shiny. Fruits like

1) Bananas
2) Strawberries
3) Gooseberries
4) Apples
5) Guavas
6) Mangoes
7) Apricots
8) Peaches
9) Watermelon

Best Nuts for your hair:

You can have for your hair.

1) Almonds
2) Walnuts
3) Figs
4) Dates
5) Kiwi

Best Vegetables for your hair:

Best vegetables to keep your hair fresh. Dark Leafy Vegetables & Salad in the morning will benefit your hair. A **spinach** leafy vegetable is best for our overall health and it suits all body types.

1) Spinach
2) Cucumber is must to add in your salad.
3) Beetroots
4) Sweet Potatoes
5) Onion
6) Carrots

Best Massage for your hair:

Oil message not only our hair need it but also the whole body needs it. It relaxes and lubricants the systems. It eases our muscles and removes pain from our body. It helps to relieve stiffness in our whole body and you can feel the overall health improvement if we make a habit to do things on regular basis. Body massage you can do in the evening.

Do Scalp Massage with **coconut** oil at night.

Massage your scalp and neck slowly with your fingers in circulation motion. After doing circular massage then do tapping massage with your finger for 2 to 3 minutes then ties your hair into braids and in morning wash it with any mild/ herbal shampoo. This process you can do alternate days or in a week 3 times. Some best hair oil for your head:

1) Coconut Oil (Whole body oil)

2) Almond Oil

3) Sesame Oil

4) Olive Oil (Whole body oil)

5) Sunflower Oil

6) Jojoba Oil

7) Peanut Oil

Best Exercises for your hair:

1. Jogging
2. Standing Fold Pose
3. Camel Pose
4. Stand and bend yourself, keep your hands on toes for 1 minute repeat this process for 5 minutes.

Acupressure Point:

(You can watch YouTube videos for Some Common Acupressure Points of hair) or press the star points which has shown in the picture mentioned below. Do the same processes which I have mentioned before i.e locate the points in your palm & stimulate (press & release).

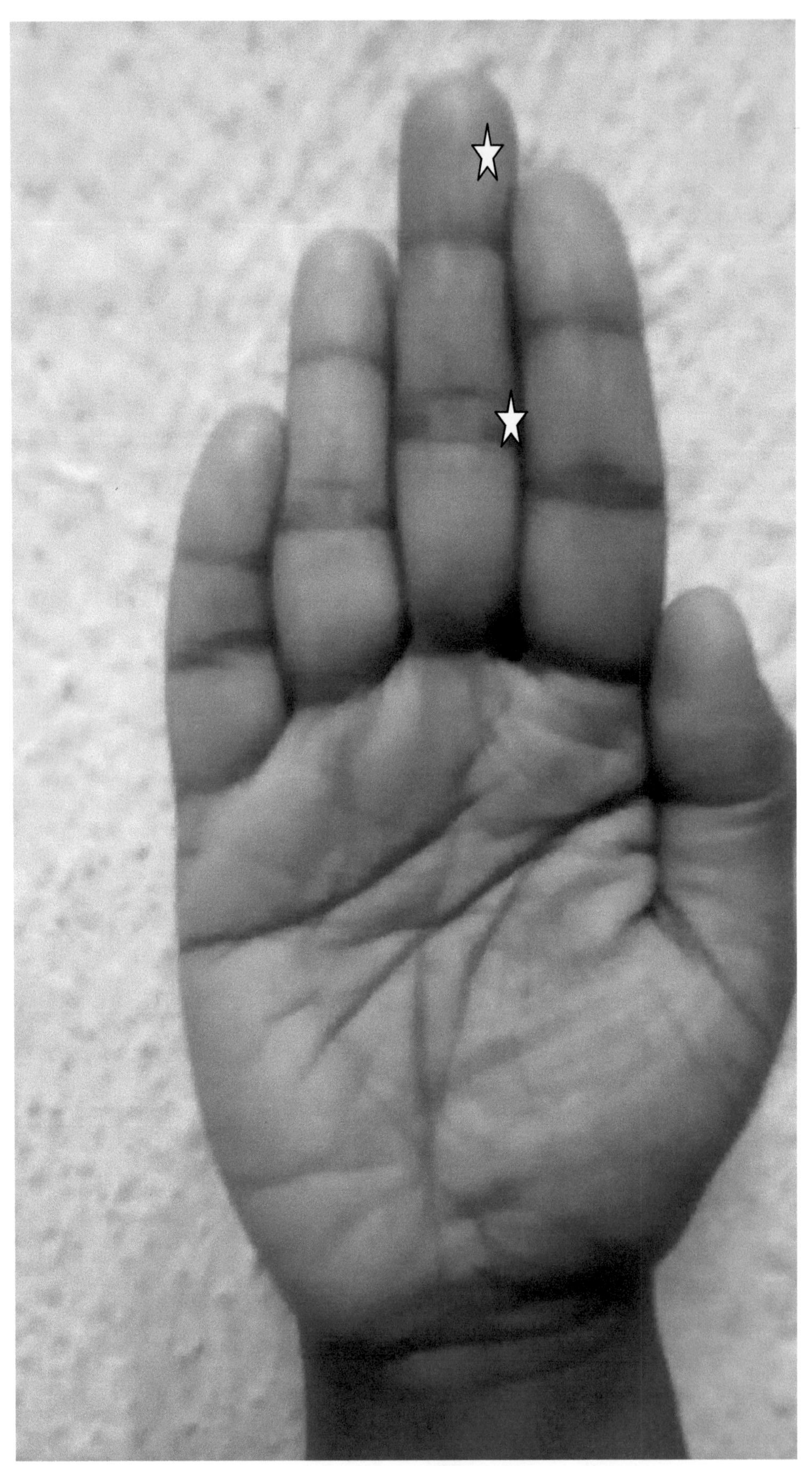

Affirm the Affirmation

Affirmation helps to control your negative thoughts!

Thank you God,

I am happy, healthy & have perfect vision of life.

Connect yourself with **God** so you will always act right at the right moment.

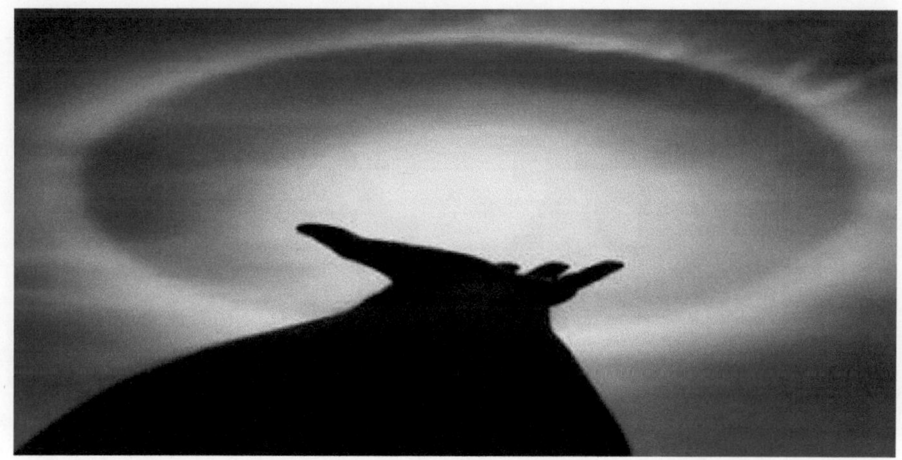

3) Skin Healthy Food

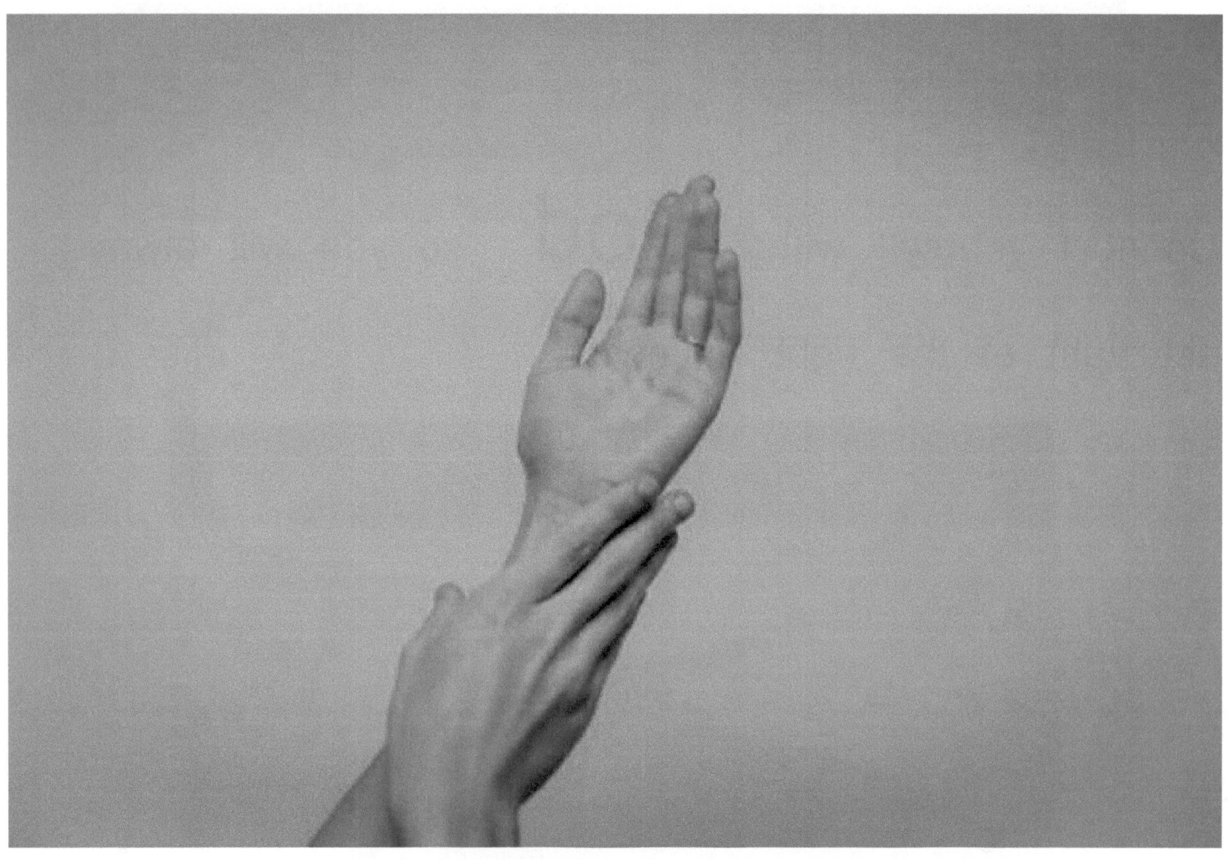

Best Fruits for your skin:

Fruit always keeps us away from any ailments.

Some Best Fruits for our body are:

1) Bananas
2) Strawberries
3) Gooseberries
4) Oranges
5) Apples
6) Guavas
7) Watermelons
8) Lemons
9) Mangoes
10) Pomegranate
11) Grapefruits
12) Pineapples.
13) Our body loves all types of berries

Sometime, we like to eat junk food but after we had, how do we feel; bad, isn't it? Yes, it affects our body and system.

When something it's not good for our body so why are we trying hard to give wrong things and sometime we force our body to take all that we wish to have for that day. This type of diet will certainly harm our body and it makes us sick.

In life, we came to this world to live happy and make others happy. So we should not try hard to eat junk food and trouble others. We are here to eat best and be best!

Best Vegetables for Skin:

1) Sweet potatoes
2) Red or yellow bell peppers
3) Broccoli
4) Tomatoes
5) Red grapes
6) Carrots.
7) Avocado
8) Spinach.

Best Massage for your skin:

Massage reduces muscle pain, relieves stress and helps you sleep better.

If you massage everyday for 5-10 minutes it helps to improve your blood circulation, tightens skin and gives fresh look every day and you will be happy to watch them.

You can try Coconut Oil for face & body massage.

Virgin Olive Oil for face & body massage.

Almond Oil for face massage.

Castor Oil for face Massage.

Best Exercises for your skin:

Exercise helps & keep your skin healthier.

1) Tapping with your fingers.
2) Kiss & Smile.
3) Puff your cheeks.
4) Lift your eyebrows

5) Make a fish face.

6) Breathing Exercises.

Acupressure Point for your skin:

(You can watch YouTube videos for Some Common Acupressure Points of skin)

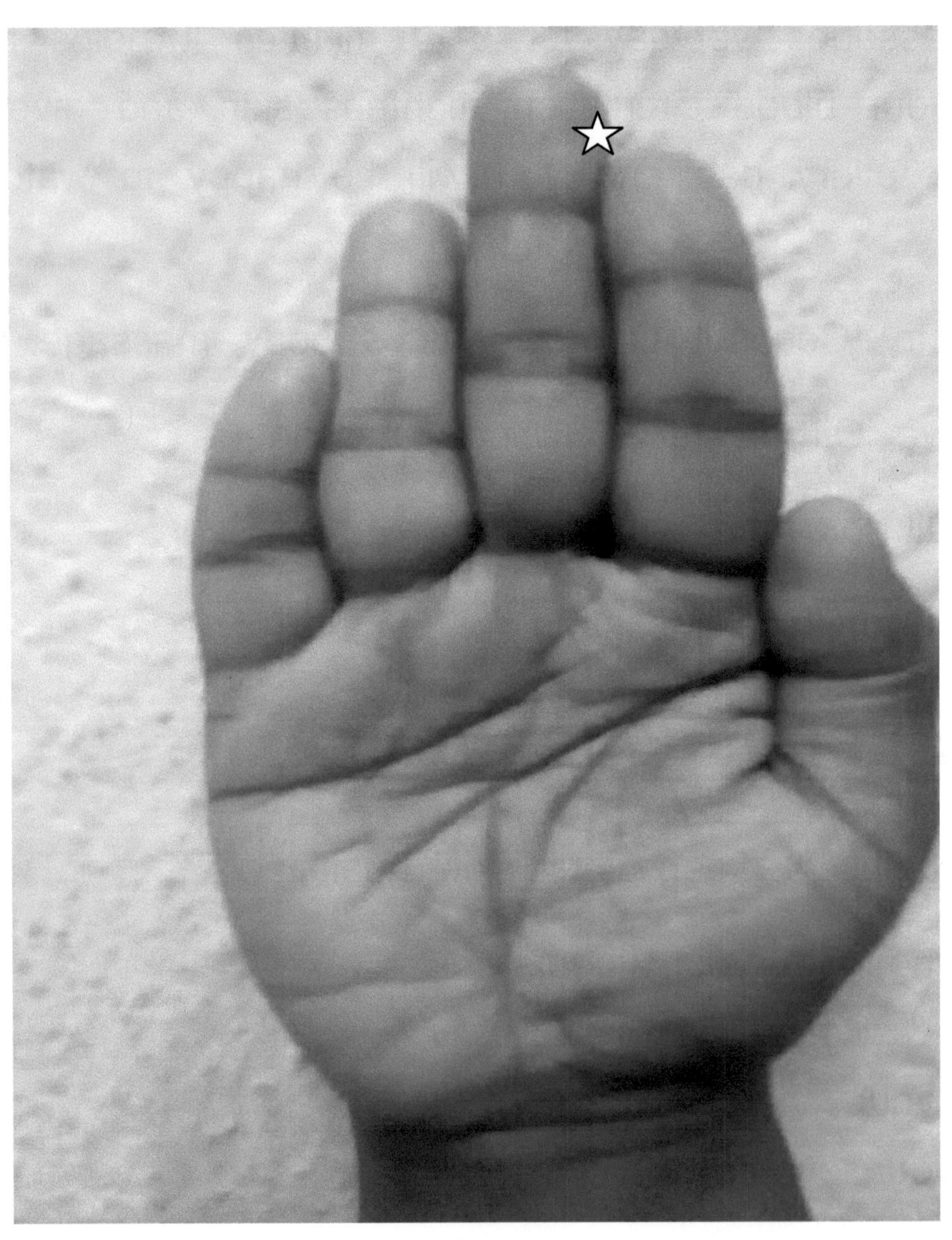

Affirm the Affirmation

Affirmation helps to control your negative thoughts!

Thank you God,

I am happy, healthy & have perfect vision of life.

Connect yourself with **God** so you will always act right at the right moment.

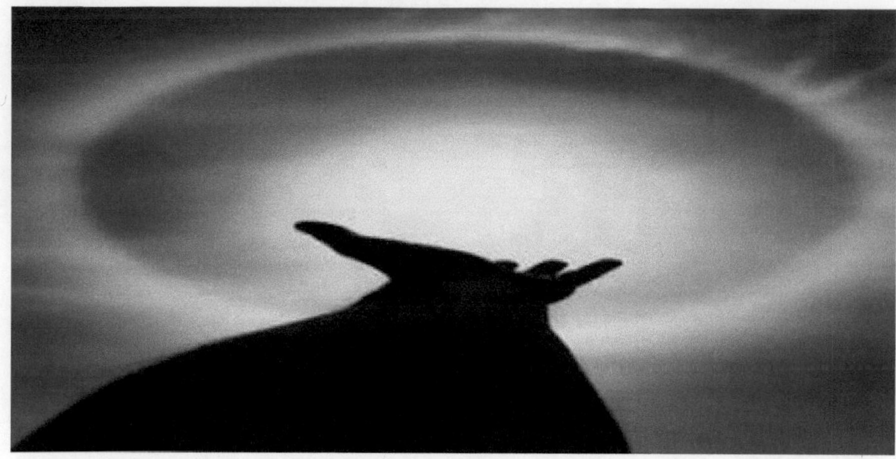

4) Bones Healthy Food

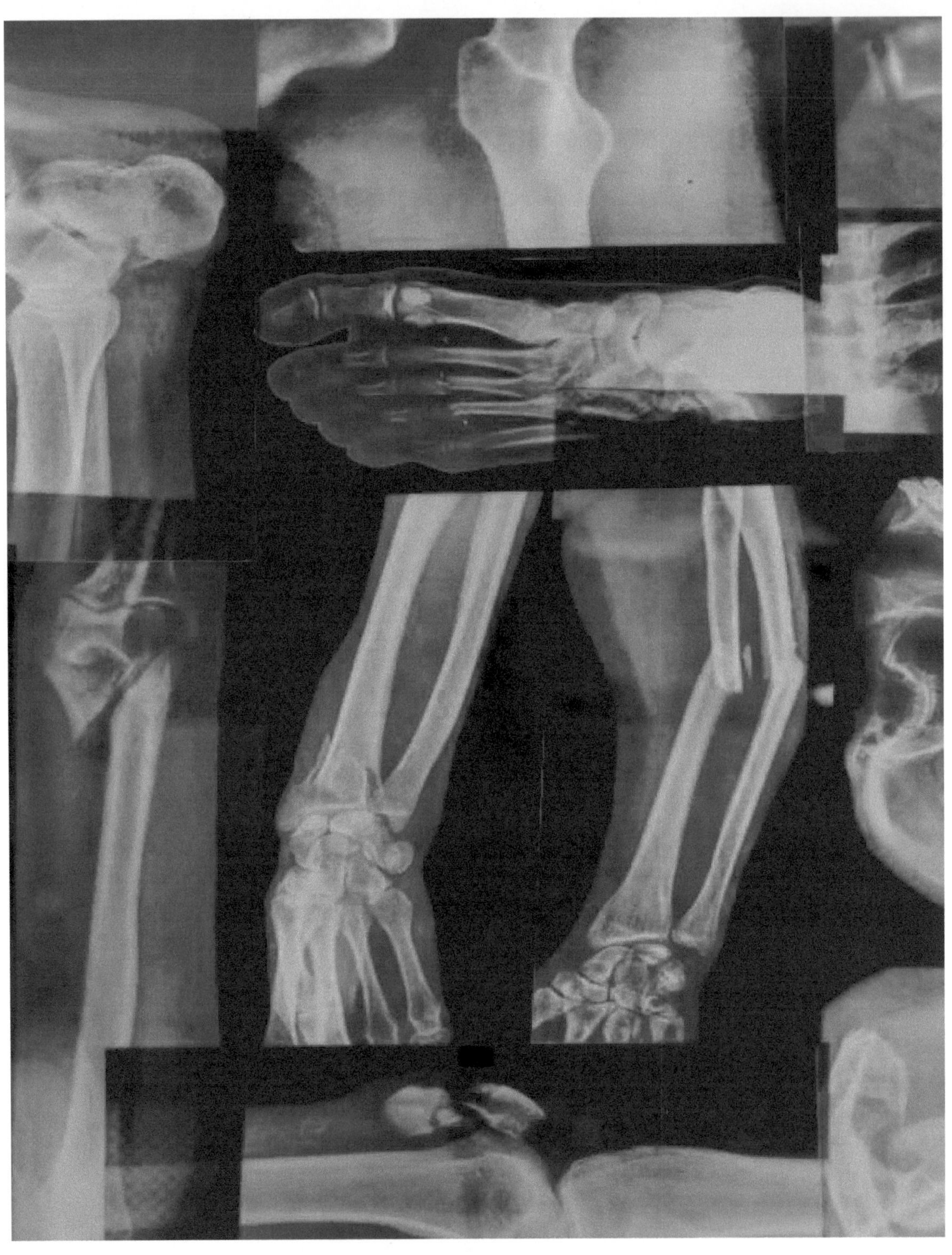

Best Fruit for bones:

If we want to keep our bones healthy it needs fruits, dark leafy vegetables, other vegetables, plant seeds, oats, nuts, cereals, pulses/legumes, water and vitamin D add to your diet that help to support strong bones and muscles. Eating foods that are rich in calcium and vitamin D is important for our bone health.

Some fruits are:

1) Pineapple
2) Strawberries
3) Oranges
4) Apples
5) Bananas
6) Guavas
7) Grape Fruit
8) Strawberries
9) Blueberries
10) Raspberries
11) Plums
12) Figs

Bones need these 2 things (Calcium & Vitamin D) to make your bones strong.

Sunlight is best source of Vitamin D.

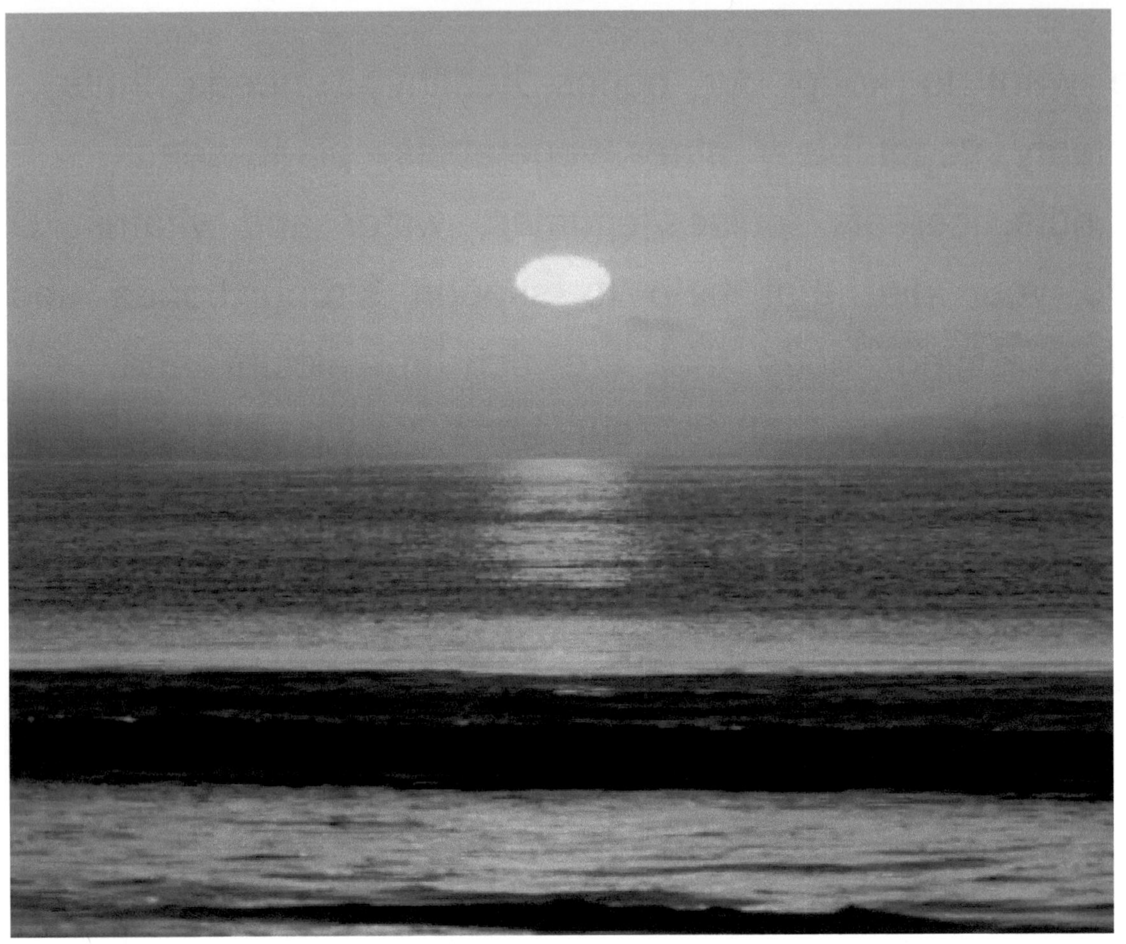

To improve your bone health please add mentioned food also in your balanced diet.

1) Milk
2) Cheese
3) Egg
4) Bone fish
5) Nuts & seeds
6) Yogurt

Best Vegetables for bones:

1) Broccoli
2) Okra
3) Dried peas
4) Beans
5) Kale
6) Dark green leafy vegetables

Best Massage Oil for bones:

Sesame oil improves the health of the body tissues and rejuvenates them. It is for everyone.

1) Sesame Oil
2) Olive Oil
3) Coconut Oil
4) Almond Oil
5) Grapes Seed Oil
6) Sunflower Oil

Massage with warm oil on your body at least for 15 minutes and leave it for 10 minutes and then go & take a bath.

Best Exercises for bones:

1) Walking
2) Jogging
3) Climbing stairs
4) Play some outdoor games

Acupressure Point for strong bones:

(You can watch YouTube videos for Some Common Acupressure Points of bones) or press the star points which has shown in the picture mentioned below.

Locate these star points on your thumb and stimulate these points, just press these points for 15 seconds and release, continue this process for 5 to 10 minutes.

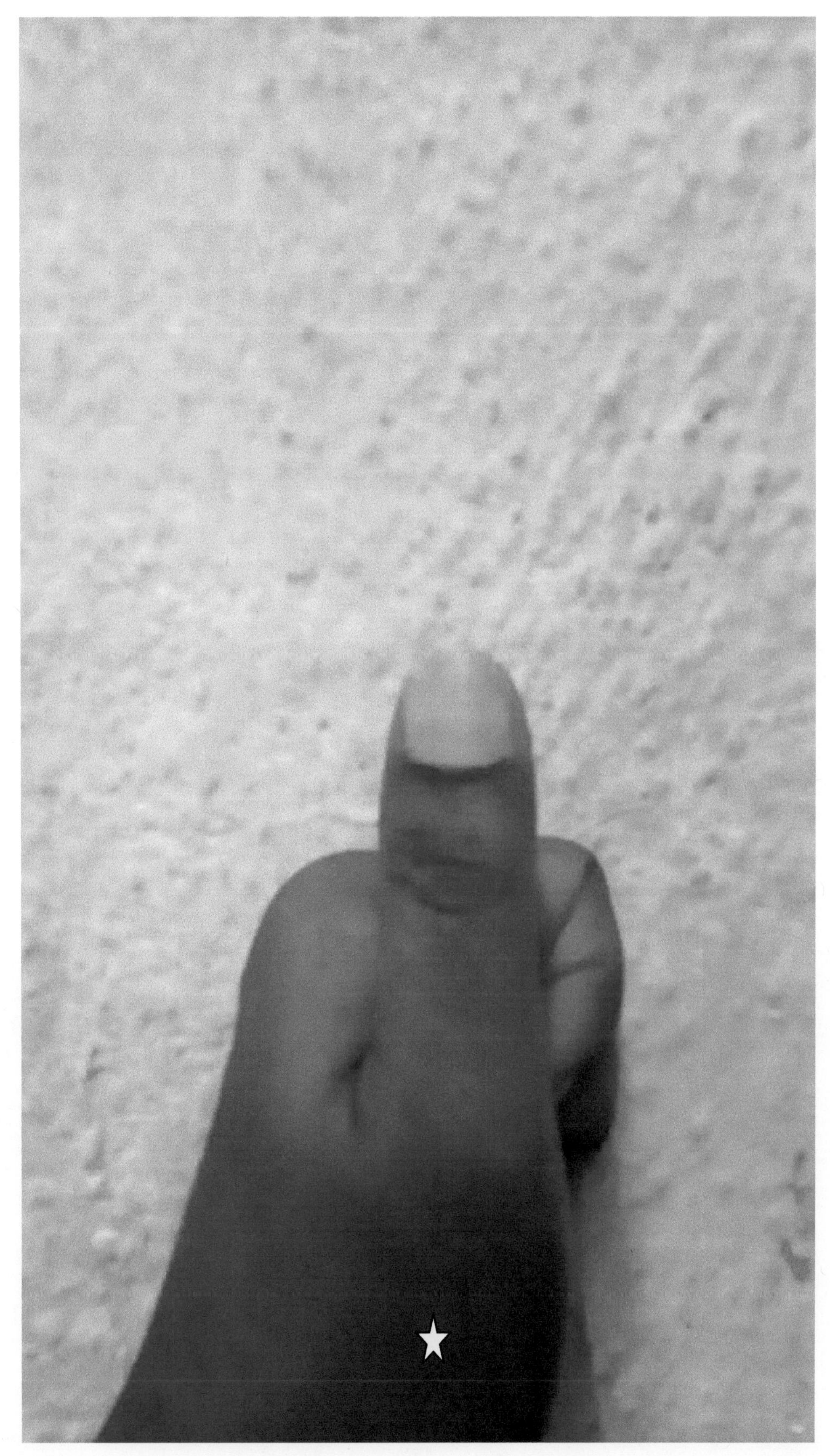

Affirm the Affirmation

Affirmation helps to control your negative thoughts!

Thank you God,

I am happy, healthy & have perfect vision of life.

Connect yourself with God so you will always act right at the right moment.

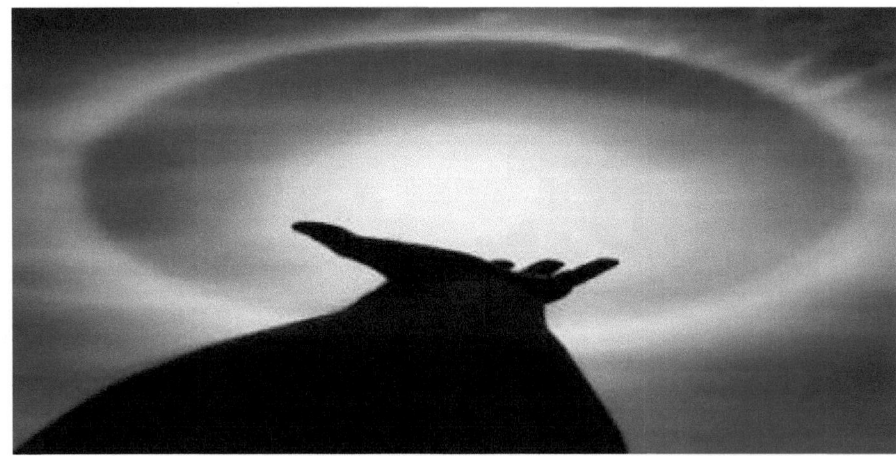

5) Stomach Healthy Food

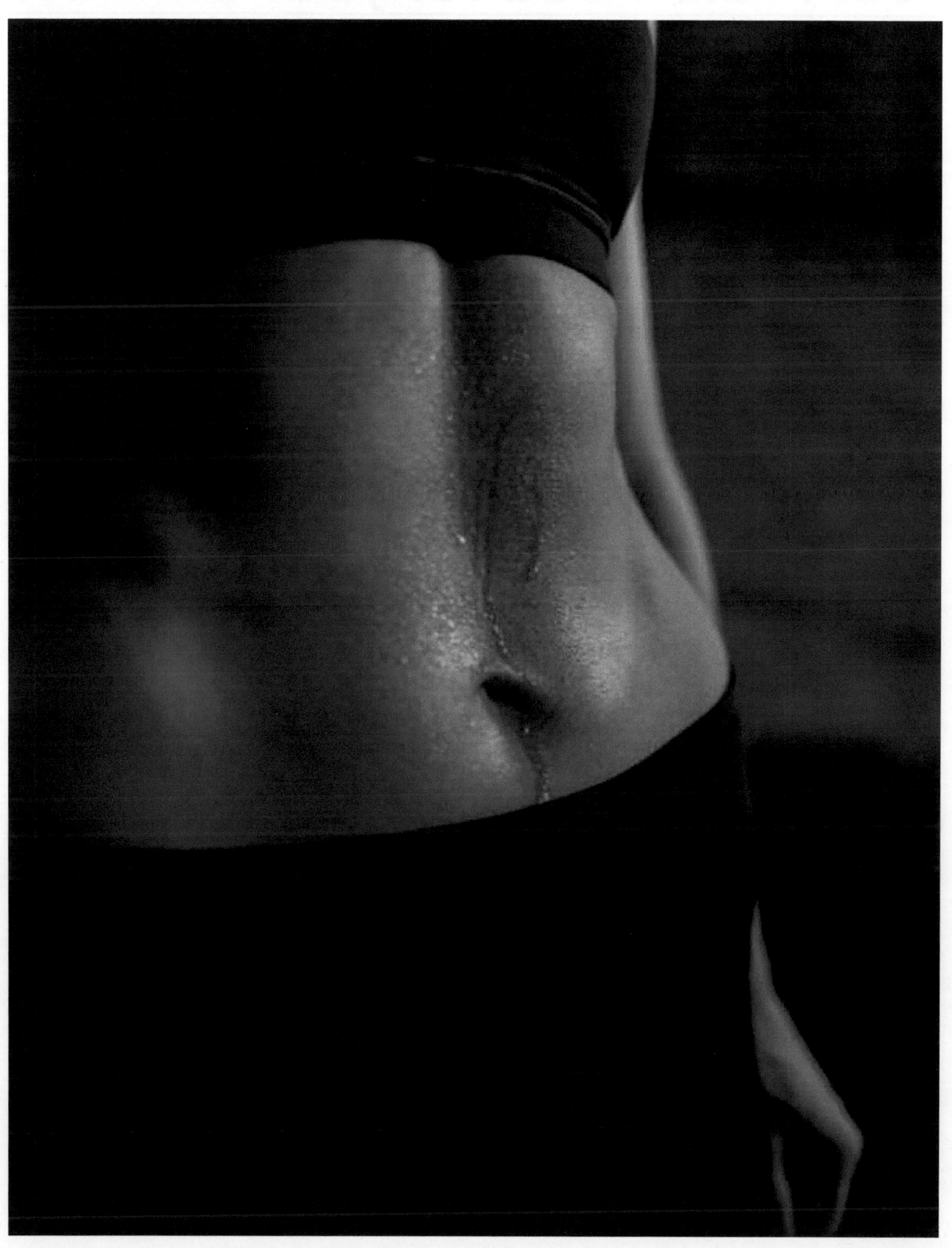

Best Fruit/ Food for your stomach, you can try:

1) Apples
2) Pears
3) Mango
4) Berries
5) Oranges
6) Grapefruit
7) Bananas
8) Berries
9) Avocados (improves your digestion)
10) Brown Rice is the best food for stomach.
11) Yogurt.
12) Honey with warm water.
13) Turmeric (a pinch of turmeric with hot water in the morning)
14) Aloe Vera Juice
15) Garlic (roast garlic)

Best Vegetables for your stomach:

1) Spinach
2) Black beans
3) Ginger
4) Leafy green vegetables
5) Sprouts
6) Broccoli
7) Cabbage
8) Cauliflower
9) Sweet potatoes
10) Pumpkin
11) Beets
12) Green beans
13) Carrots
14) Bitter gourd
15) Cucumber
16) Drum Stick

Best Massage for your stomach:

Stomach massage can help to cleanse your body. It also help to relieve symptoms of tightness, acidity or bloating, cramping. To massage start from the right to left, in a clockwise motion.

Best Exercises for your stomach:

1) You can start by lying down flat with your knees bent and your feet touch on the ground.
2) Walking
3) Running.
4) Swimming.
5) Cycling.

Acupressure Point for your stomach:

(You can watch YouTube videos for Some Common Acupressure Points of stomach) or press the star points which has shown in the picture mentioned below.

Locate these star points on your palm and stimulate these points, just press these points for 10 seconds and release, simultaneously do breathe in & breathe out. Please repeat the process for 5 to 10 minutes.

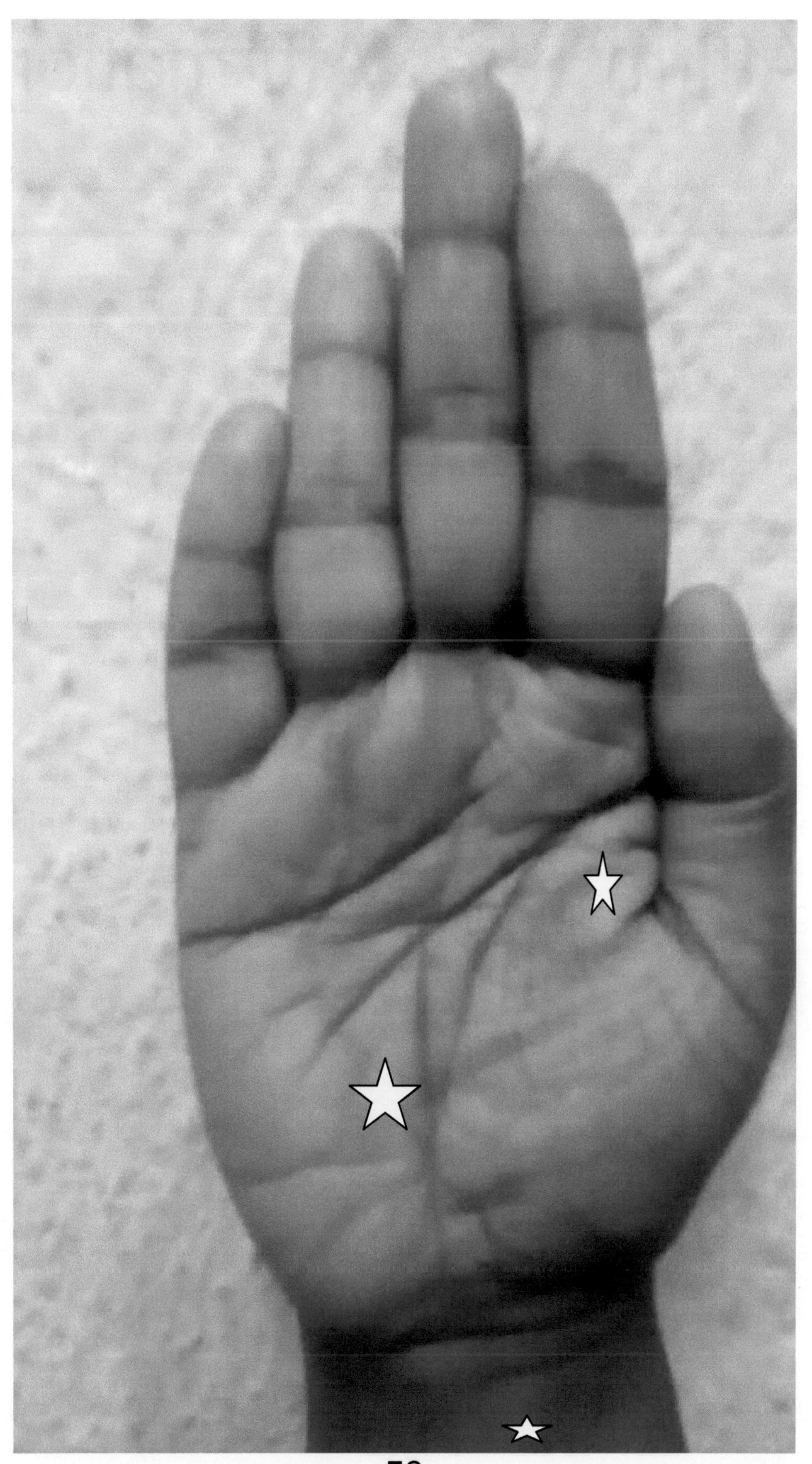

Affirm the Affirmation

Affirmation helps to control your negative thoughts!

Thank you God,

I am happy, healthy & have perfect vision of life.

Connect yourself with God so you will always act right at the right moment.

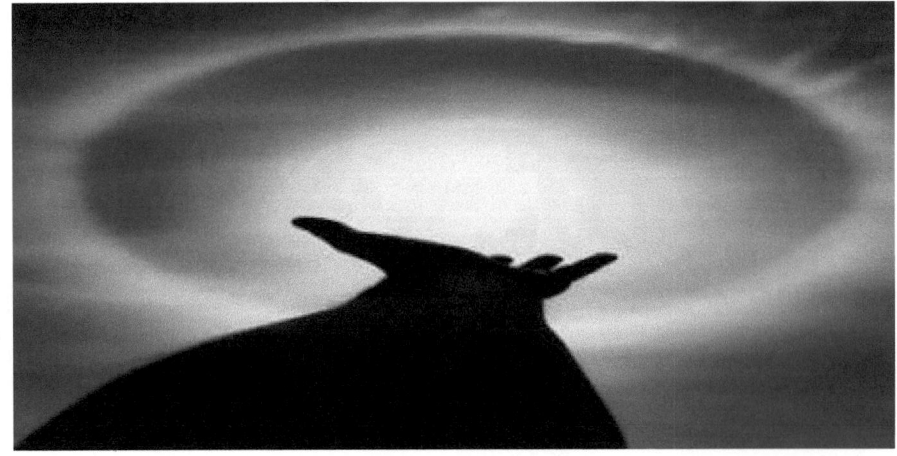

6) Heart Healthy Food

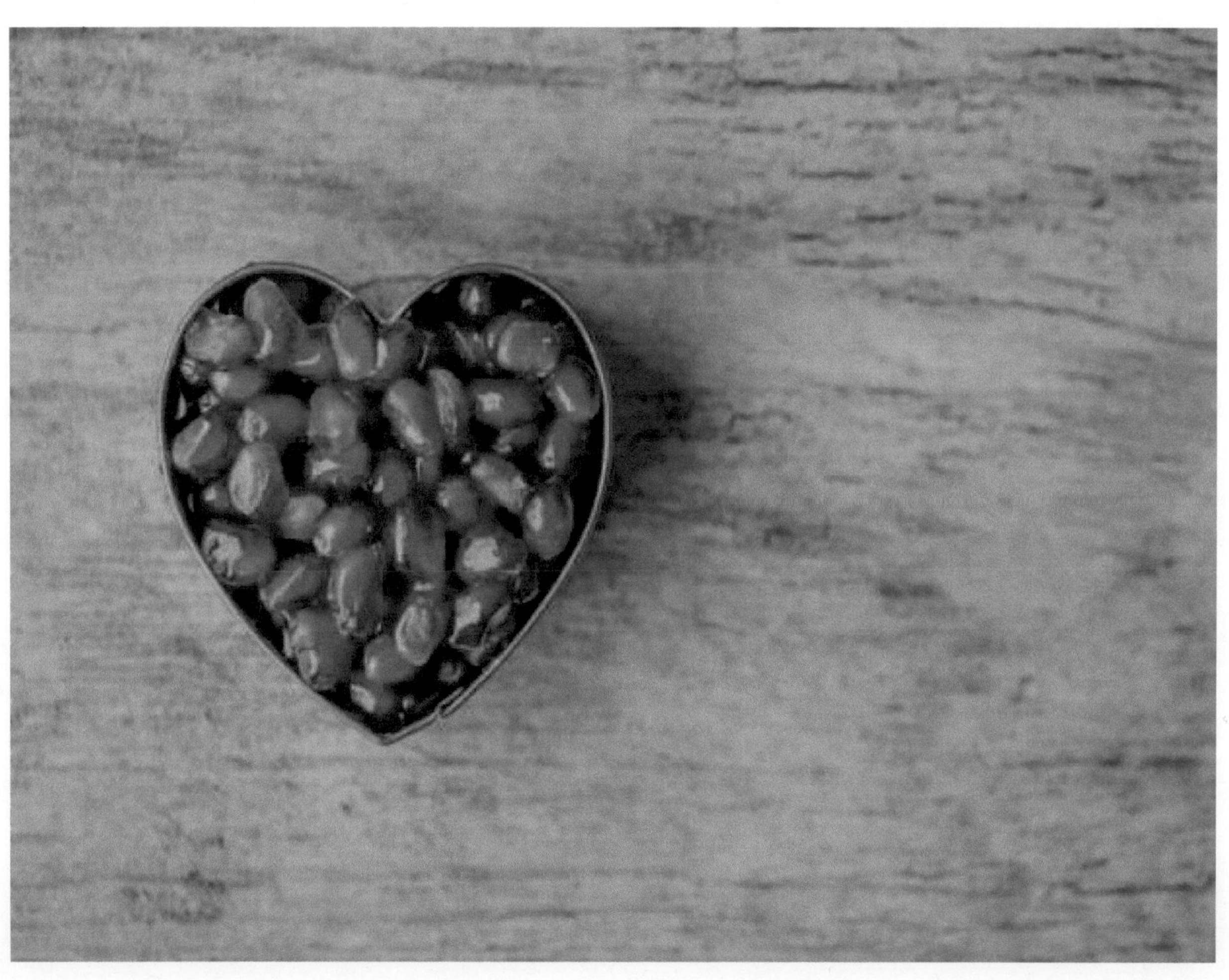

Heart loves chocolate so you can have chocolate.

Best Fruit for your heart:

1. Watermelon
2. Strawberries
3. Blueberries
4. Blackberries
5. Raspberries
6. Avocados
7. Banana

Best Vegetables for your heart:

1. Broccoli
2. Kale
3. Sprouts
4. Tomatoes
5. Bell Peppers
6. Carrots
7. Beans
8. Beetroot
9. Cucumber

Best Nuts for your heart:

1. Walnuts
2. Almonds
3. Pistachios
4. Peanuts
5. Cashews

Best Exercises for your heart:

1) Breathe in & breathe out
2) Walking.
3) Hands up, Hands down, Hands on side
4) Rub your palm
5) Clap your hands
6) Open & Close your arms

Best Massage for your heart:

Just close your eyes; touch both of your hands close to heart and slowly do breathe in & breathe out 5 to 7 times, you will feel more relax.

Acupressure Point for your heart:

(You can watch YouTube videos for Some Common Acupressure Points of heart) or press the star points which has shown in the picture mentioned below.

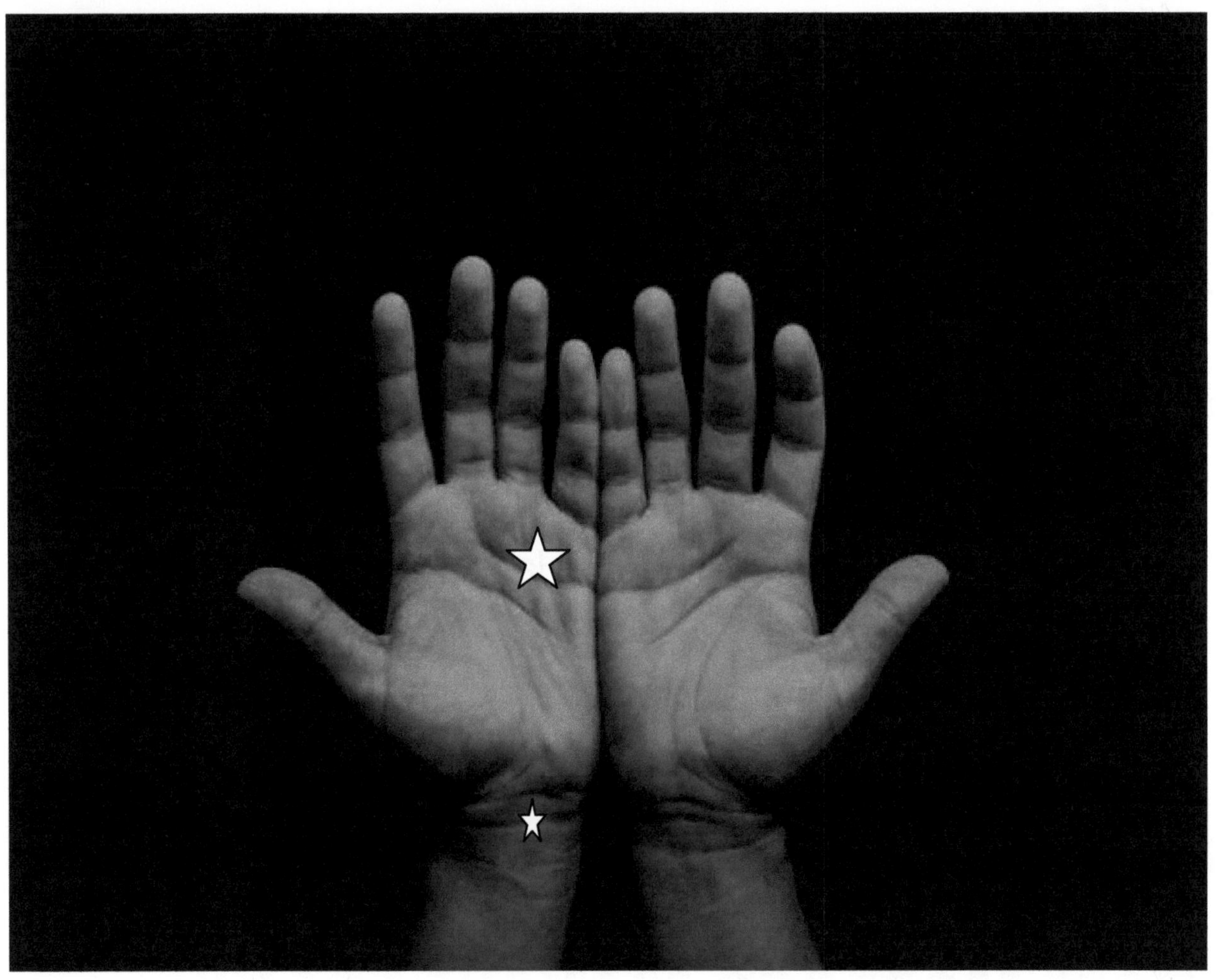

Locate these star points on your palm and stimulate these points, just press these points for 10 seconds and release, simultaneously do breathe in & breathe out. Please repeat the process for 5 to 10 minutes.

Affirm the Affirmation

Affirmation helps to control your negative thoughts!

Thank you God,

I am happy, healthy & have perfect vision of life.

Connect yourself with **God** so you will always act right at the right moment.

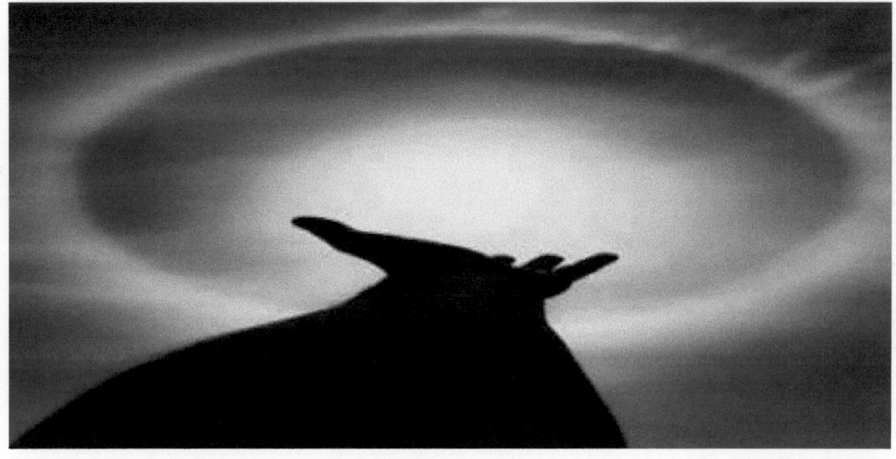

7) Muscles Best Food

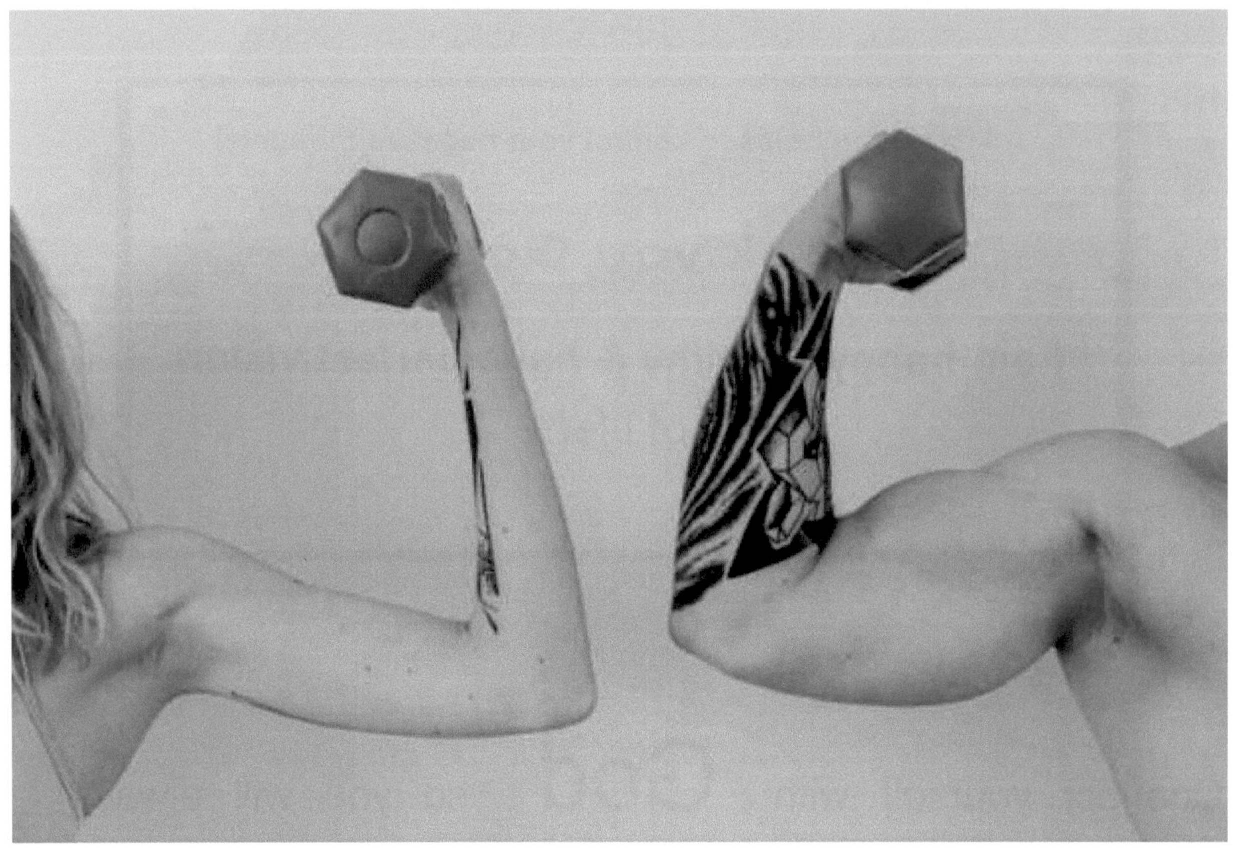

Some best fruits for muscle building.

Best Fruit for muscles:

1. Bananas
2. Dates
3. Raisins
4. Apricots
5. Golden Raisins
6. Jackfruit

7. Avocados
8. Guavas

Along with fruits & vegetables, Poultry & Non vegetarian food is also very helpful to build muscle mass fast.

1. Eggs
2. meat
3. Fish

Best Vegetables for muscles:

1. Dark leafy vegetables
2. Peas
3. Spinach
4. Kale
5. Broccoli

Best Massage for muscles:

Massage therapy relaxes muscle tissues.

Hot stone massage is best for people who have muscle pain or who just want to relax.

Best Exercises for muscles:

1) Pushups
2) Pull-ups
3) Shoulder press

Acupressure Point for back muscles:

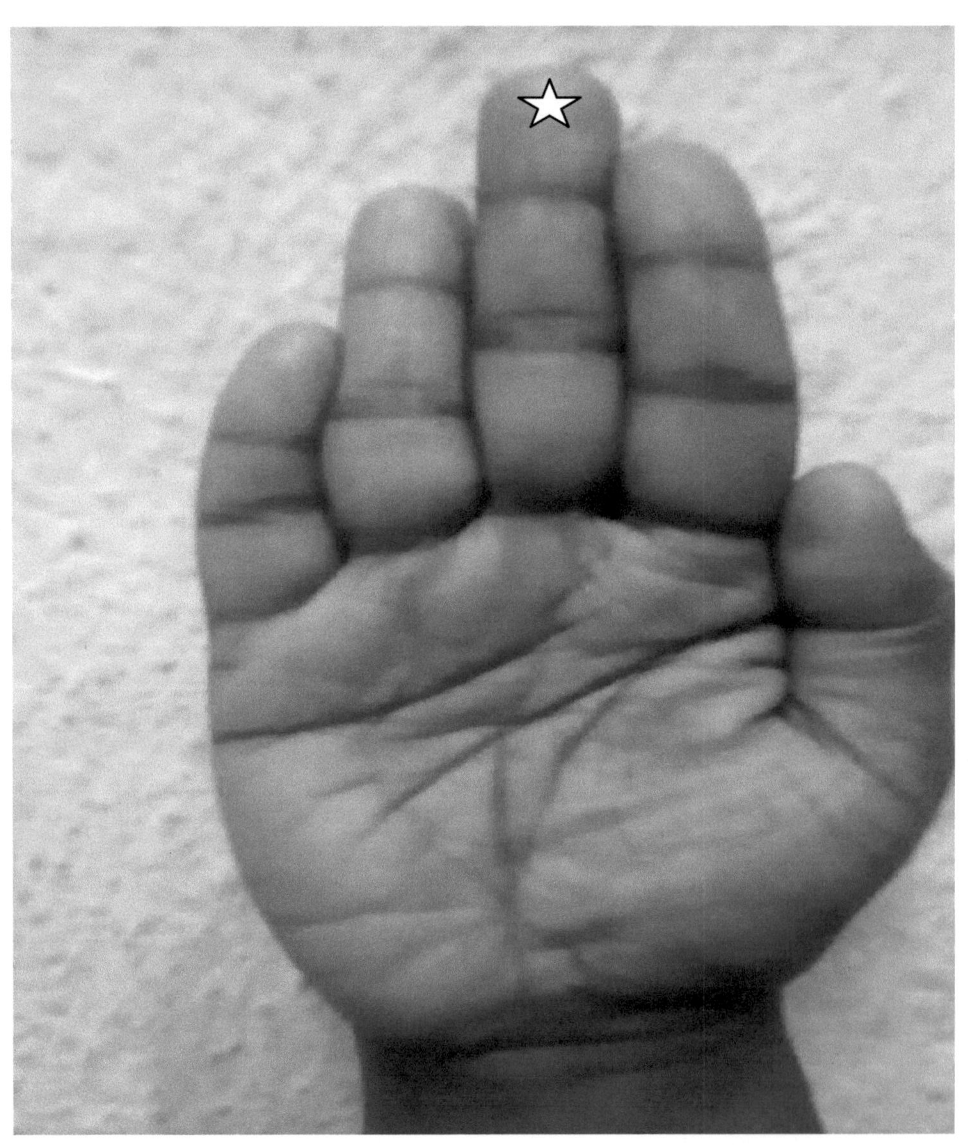

Affirm the Affirmation

Affirmation helps to control your negative thoughts!

Thank you God,

I am happy, healthy & have perfect vision of life.

Connect yourself with God so you will always act right at the right moment.

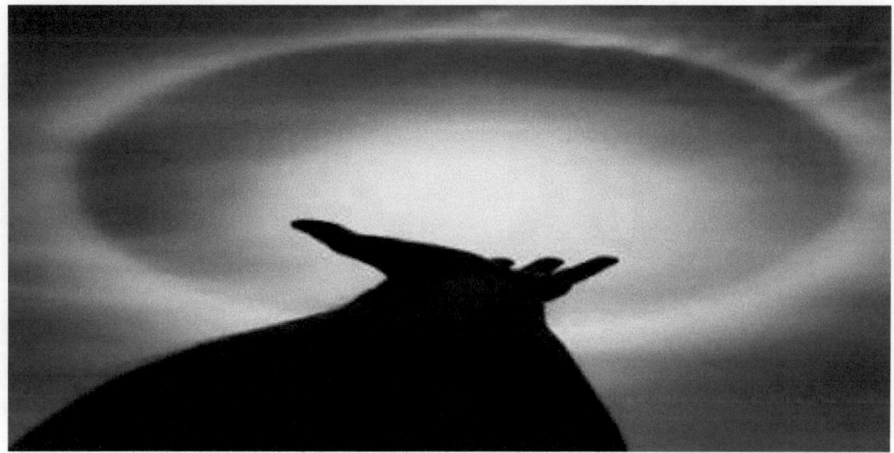

I feel if we follow all the above steps on regular basis. Most of our health related issues we face in our day to day life will end soon and we can live healthy & wonderful life till we are alive in this world.

Next, **Cleanliness**

Clean body & clean home both play an important role to be healthy & happy. When you clean your house, clean every corner of the room, entry of sunlight is important in our body as well as for our beautiful house, makes sure all the rooms are well ventilated.

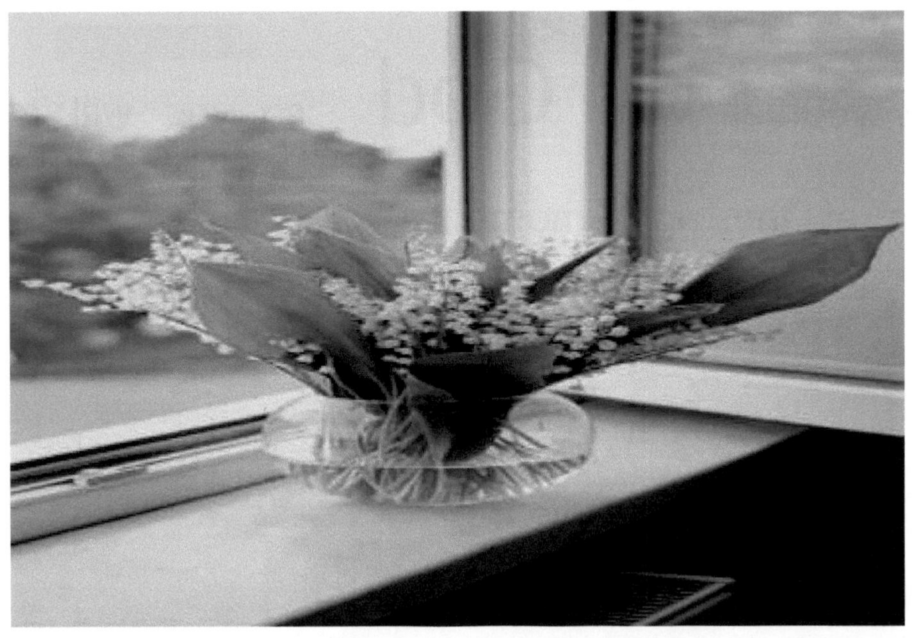

First make sure, when you are sick, keep your surrounding and yourself clean. The environment you stay in that should give you fresh & ventilated air so automatically your body vibration will change and you will soon feel fresh & heal yourself.

Follow these habits in your daily life.

1. **Brush your teeth in the morning and at bedtime.**
2. **Have a bath daily.**
3. **Keep your nails and hair clean.**
4. **Wear clean clothes.**
5. **Comb your hair.**
6. **Wash your hands after visiting the toilet.**
7. **Rinse your mouth after eating food.**
8. **Wear clean night-clothes.**
9. **Keep the environment dust free.**
10. **Do smudging with incense stick, bay leaves, Benzoin (Loban), camphor, Azadirachta Indica (neem leaves) etc.**

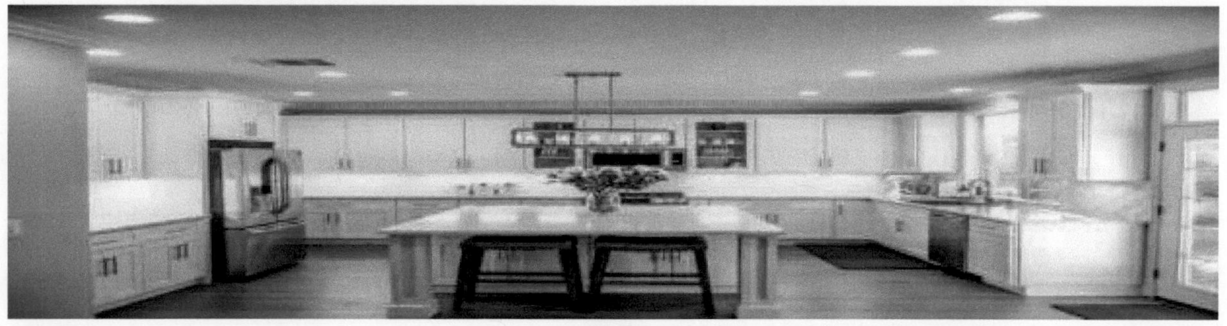

Don't forget to affirm & connect with God.

Affirm the Affirmation

Affirmation helps to control your negative thoughts!

Thank you God,

I am happy, healthy & have perfect vision of life.

Connect yourself with God so you will always act right at the right moment.

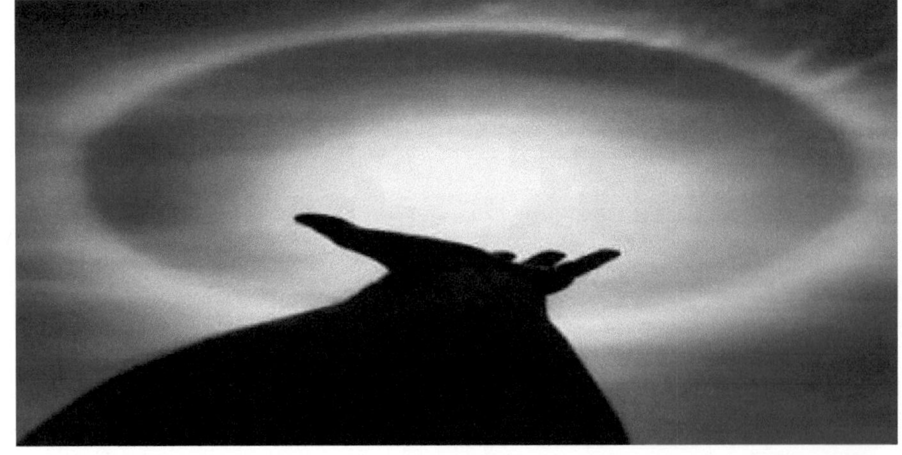

Next, Purification & Detoxification

Kidney organ in our body play a role of **purification**, it purifies our blood.

Liver: The organ Liver, it removes waste from our body i.e. **detoxification**.

Best food for Kidney & Liver.

Water

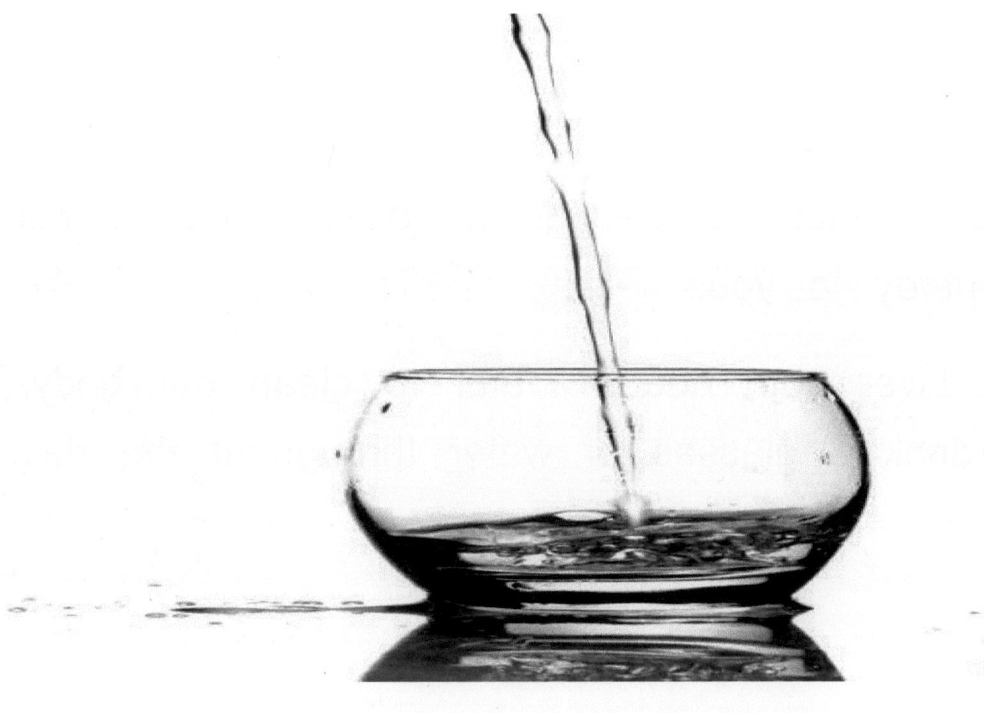

The best diet for preventing heart disease is that we should have our diet full of fruits and vegetables, whole grains, nuts, fish.

Drink: Water, Plain water is the best thing to drink for overall health, if we make a habit to drink water sip by sip early in the morning at 5 AM, it will show great health benefits.

Your kidneys depend on water because water keeps your blood vessels open so that blood can move freely.

The kidney is responsible for the purification of blood. Detoxification: Our Liver (detox manager) remove waste from our blood and it helps to convert our food to energy.

So be careful; what are you giving to your liver it will give that energy to you.

Kidney and Liver both needs Water to clean our body. So please drink 8 glasses of water throughout the day **sip by sip.**

Best Fruits for Kidney :

1) Pineapple
2) Blueberries
3) Cranberries
4) Grapefruit
5) Apples

Best Vegetables for Kidney:

1. Broccoli
2. Cabbage
3. Cauliflower
4. Sprouts
5. Garlic
6. Ginger
7. Turnip
8. Coriander leaves

You can also add Fish in your diet.

***List of Vegetables & fruits are shared based on my search, so please select your choice of fruits & vegetables that suit you the best & for your body.**

Affirmation

Affirmation helps to control your negative thoughts!

Thank you God,

I am happy, healthy & have perfect vision of life.

Connect yourself with **God** so you will always act right at the right moment.

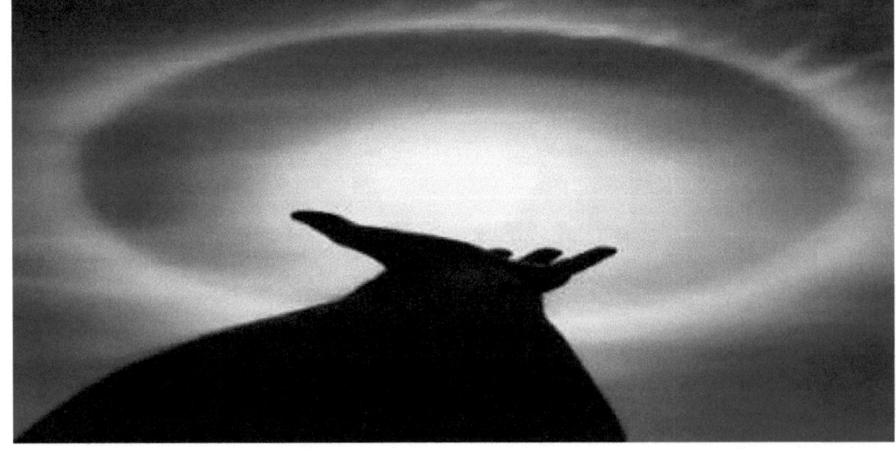

Common Problems with Quick Solution:

Giddiness: First have sugar or honey or chocolate or sugar candy, next let the person relax their whole body on floor and someone can hold both legs upside for 20 seconds and then keep the legs down repeat the process and simultaneously stimulate the acupressure point. (Check YouTube Videos) and make sure you should keep your stomach clean.

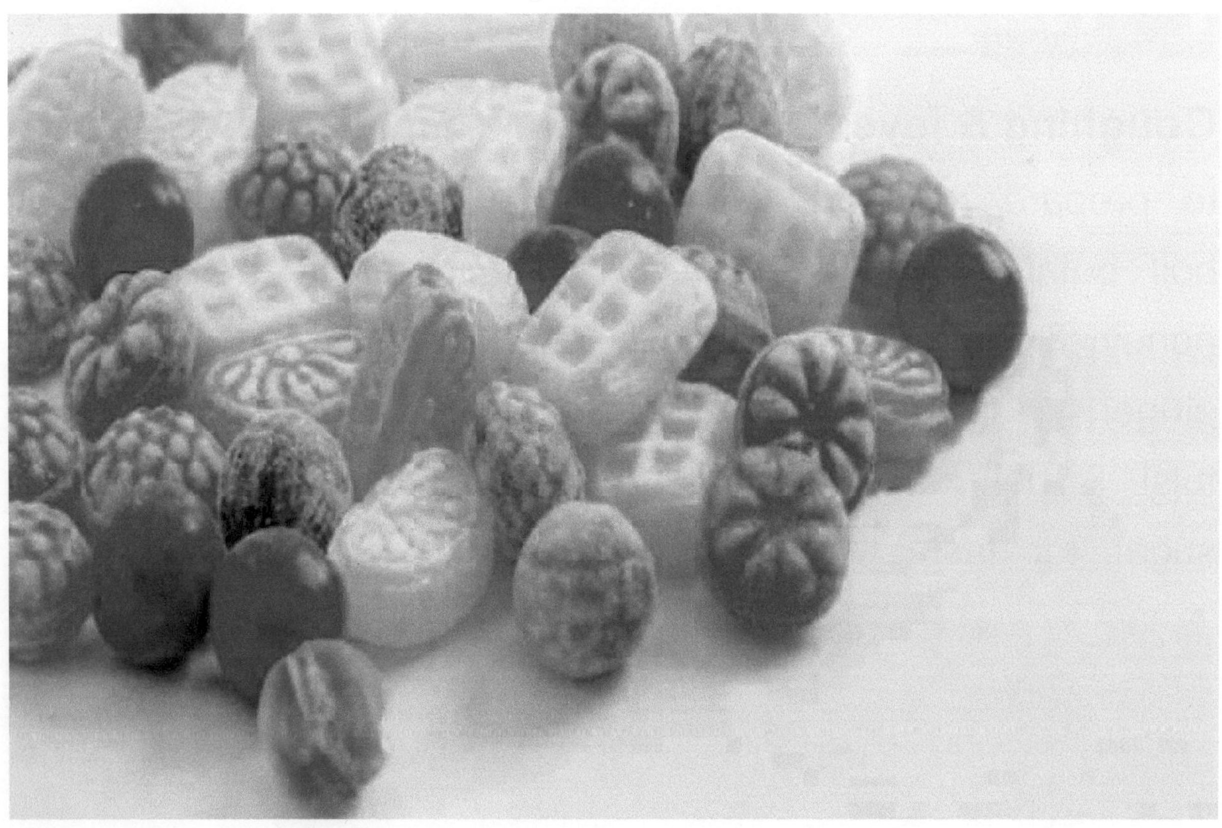

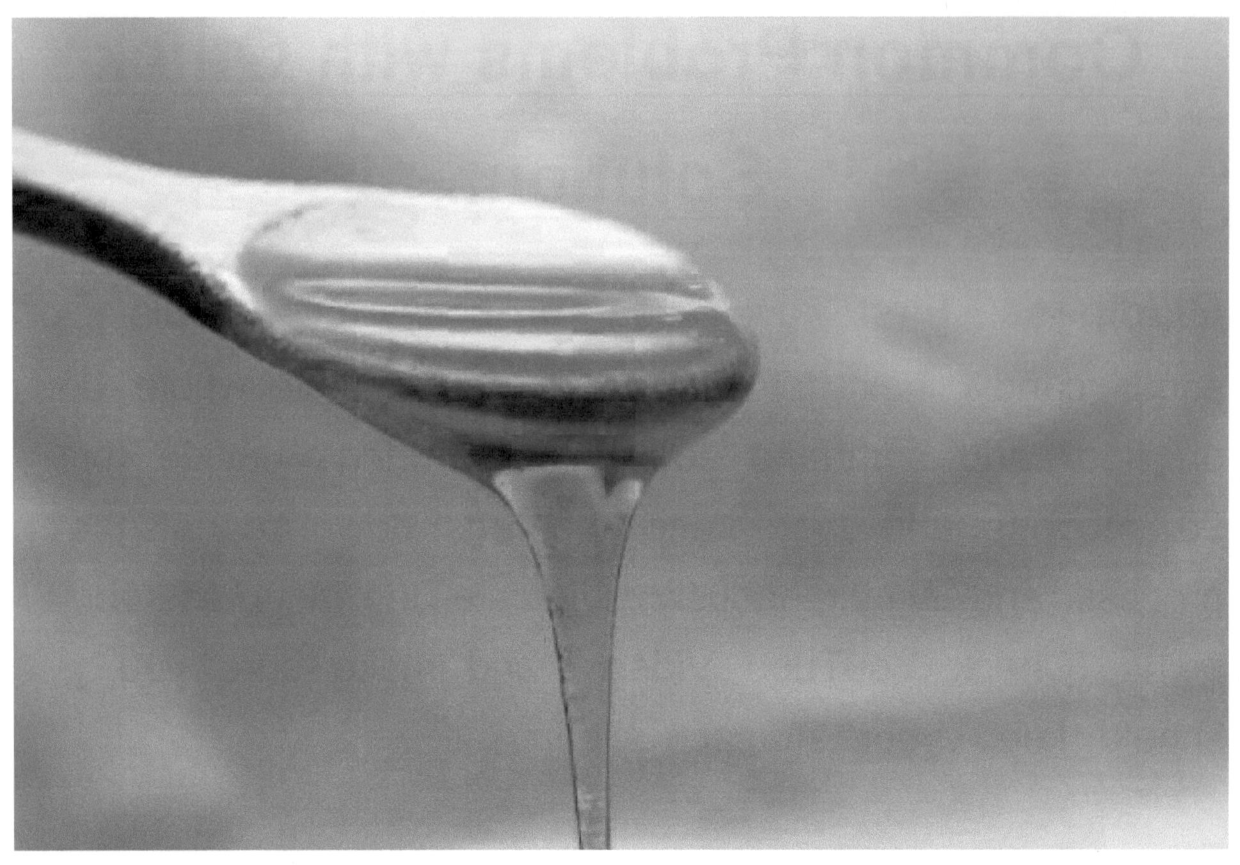

Coughing & fever: First do steaming, then prepare tea, to prepare tea add Tulsi /Basil leaves & Bel leaves boil both leaves together for 15 minutes then add honey & have it. You can also add 1 pinch of dry ginger, 1 tsp of black pepper, dry coriander seeds with tulsi & bel leaves for 15 minutes, (you can add candy sugar for taste) strain & drink.

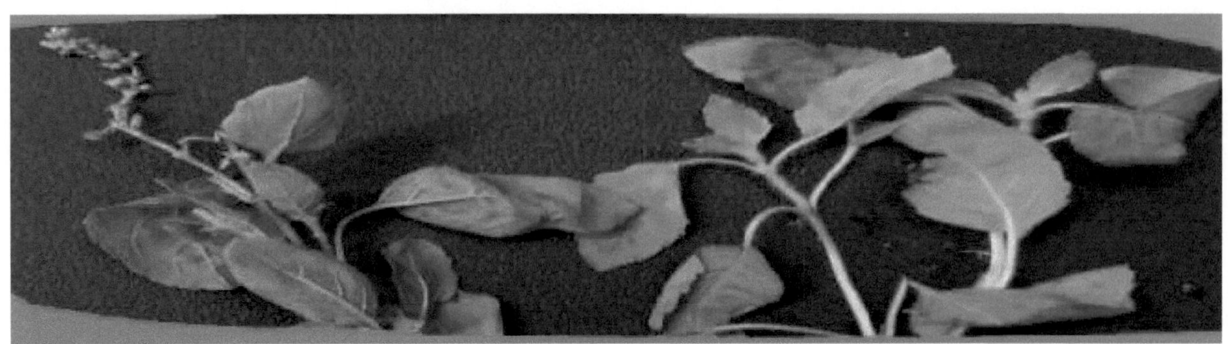

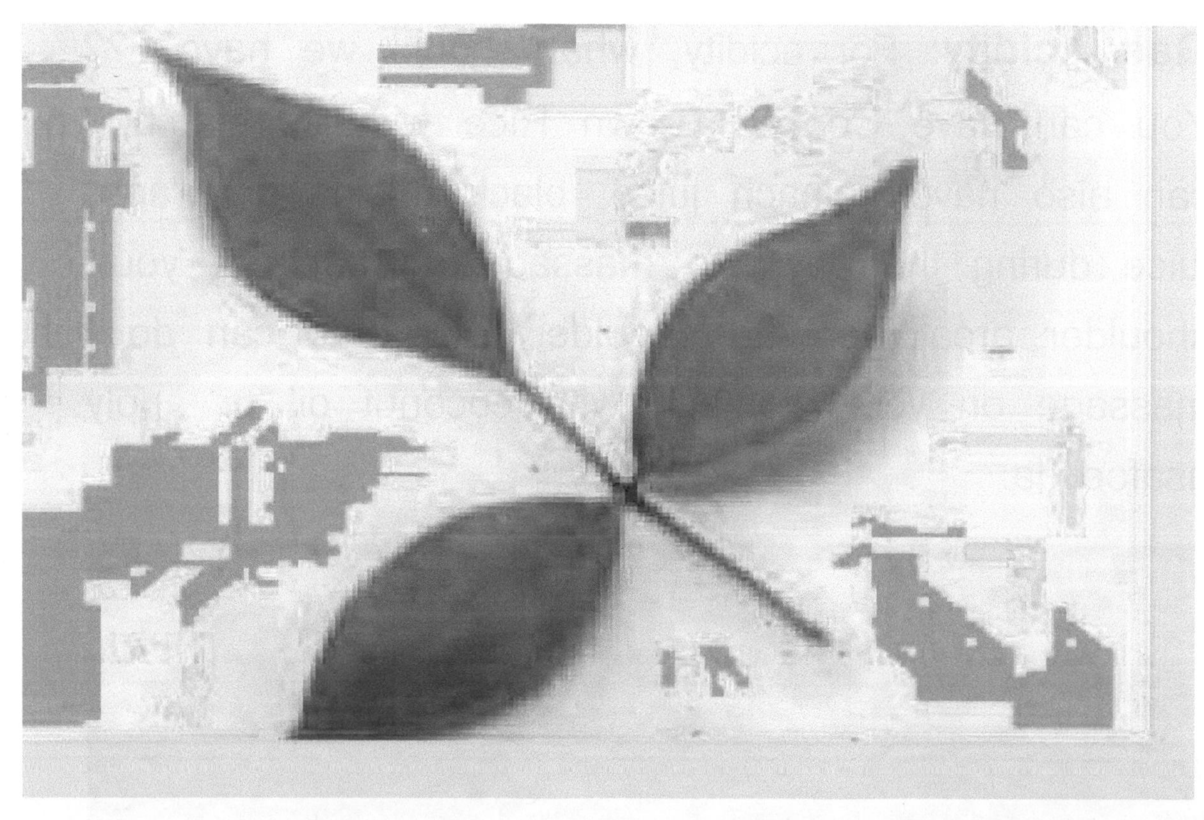

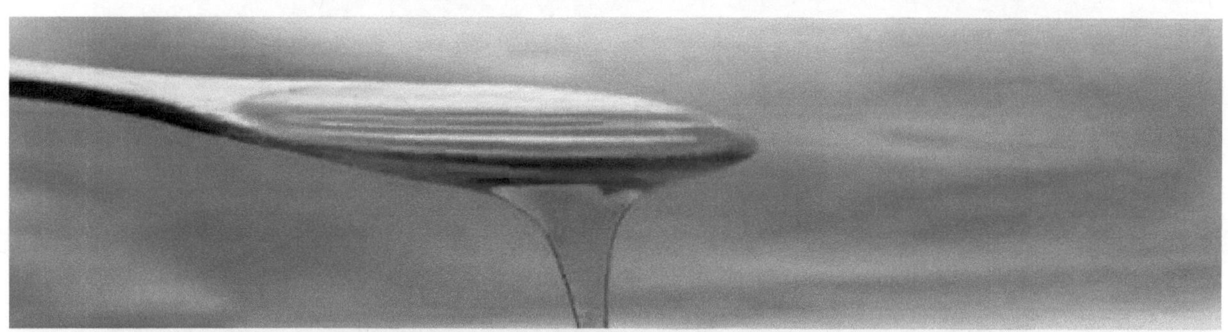

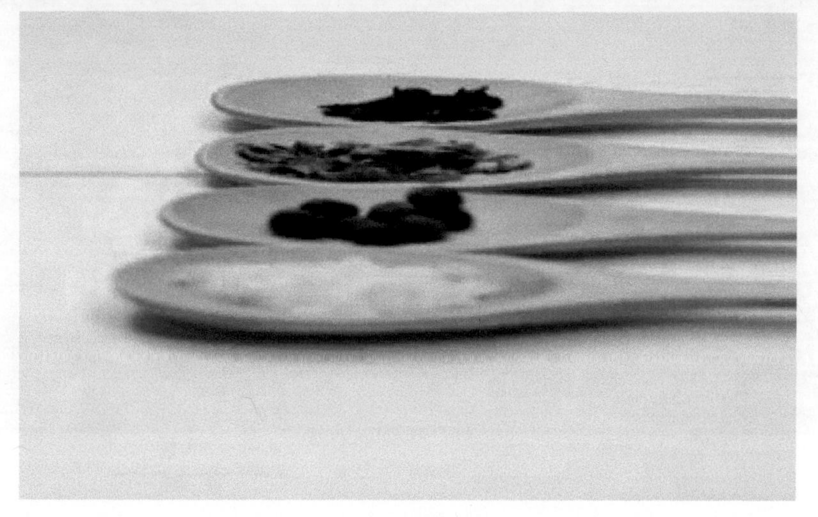

Gas/ Acidity: For acidity, what should we have???? You can have Cooked Brown Rice with its starch; you can also have spinach juice, black raisins or grapes juice during the day. Do massage on back of your shoulder area (neck to shoulder) also you can do light massage on your stomach with coconut oil or apply asafoetida.

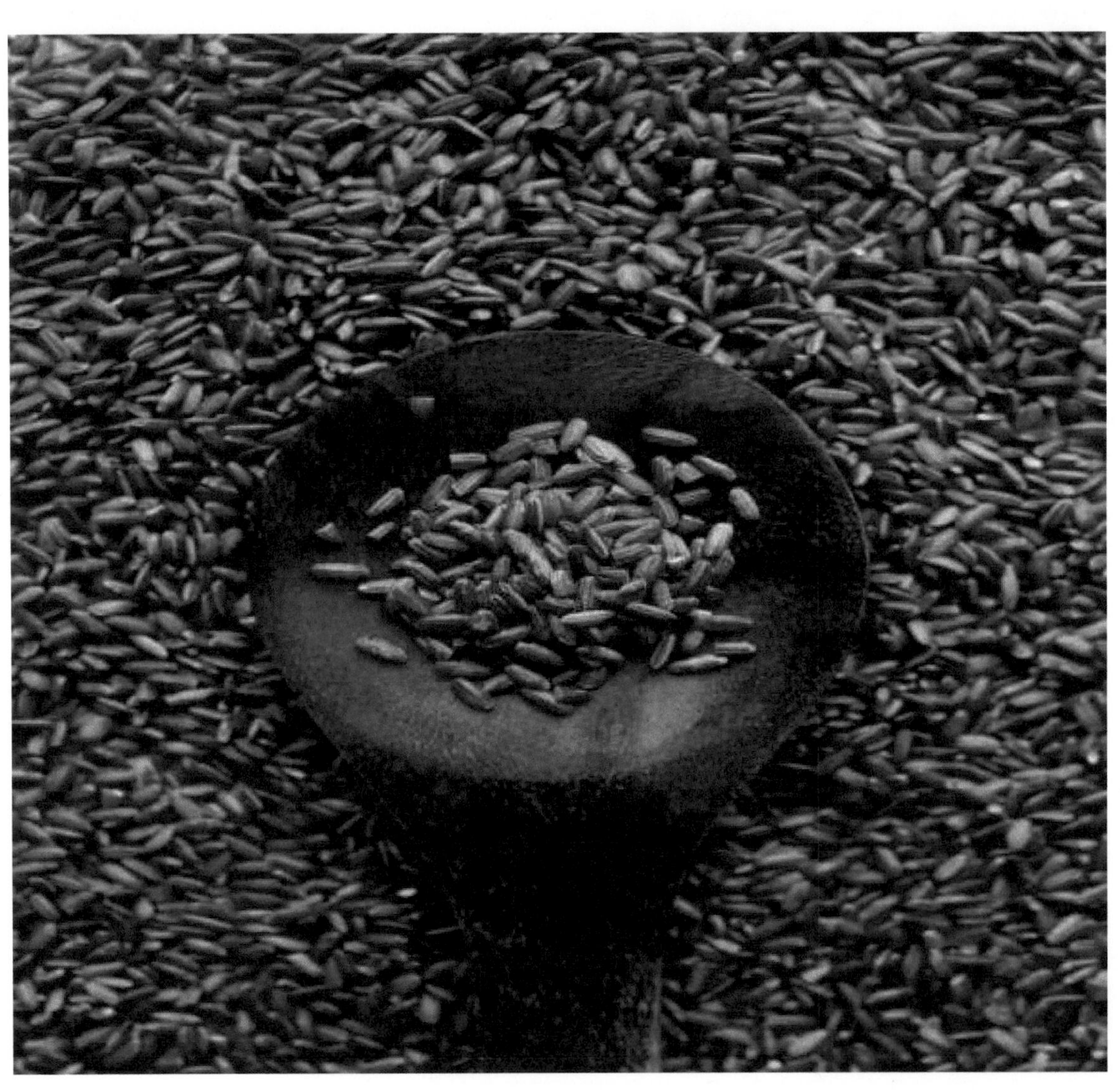

Vomiting: Orange juice, sweet lime juice, coconut water, dry black raisins are some of best juices you can try.

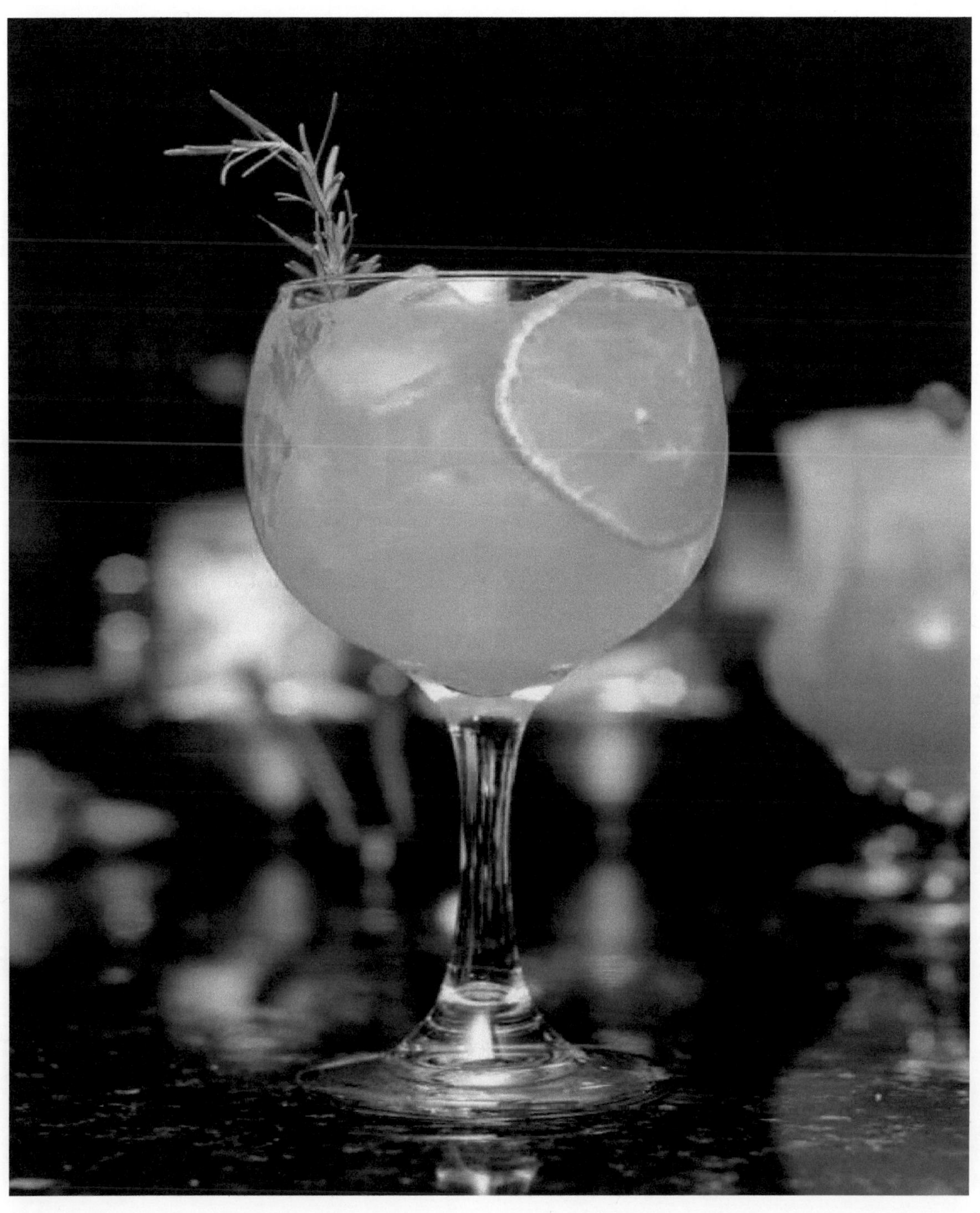

Loose motion: Have lemon juice or lick lemon juice.

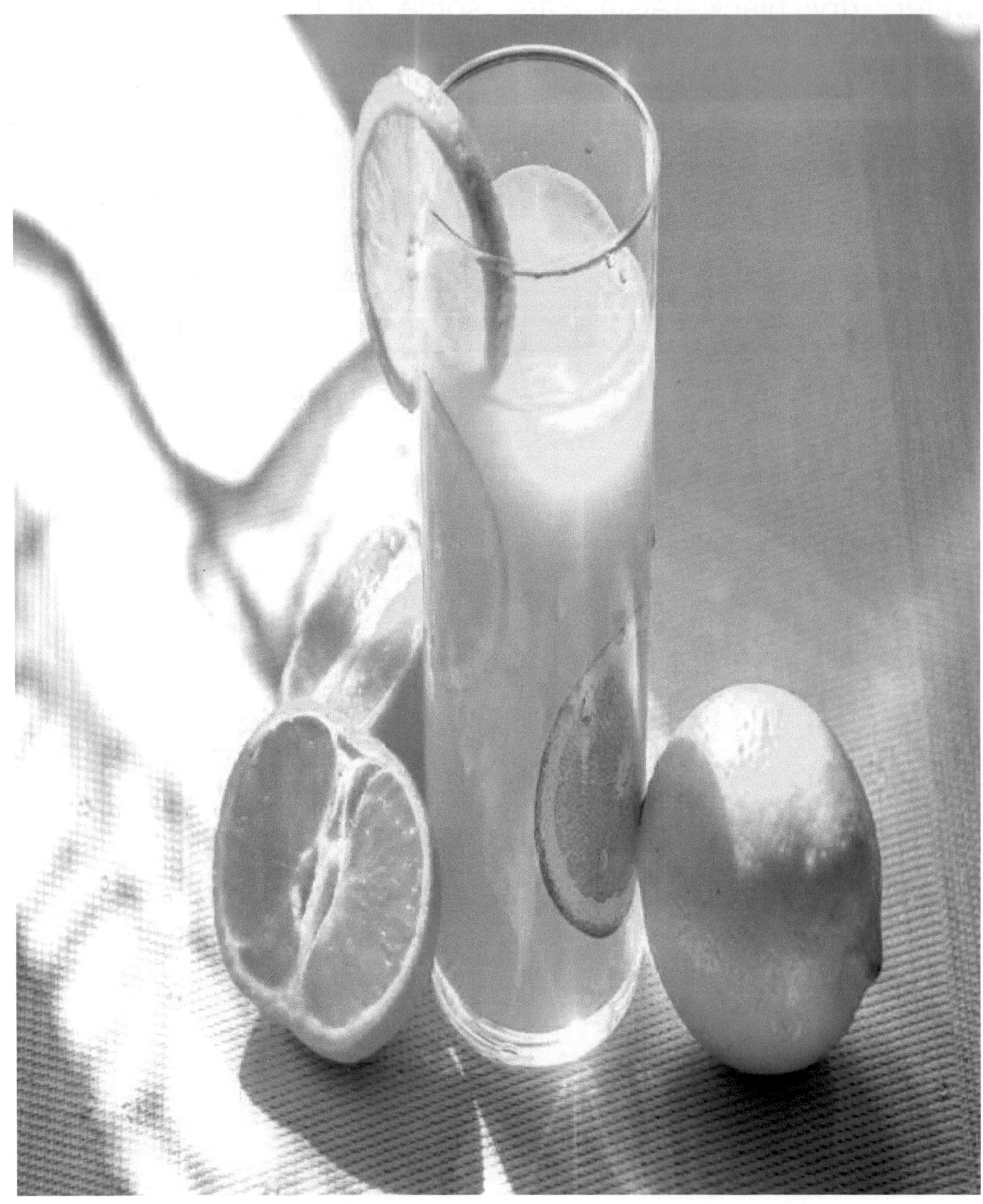

Constipation: For constipation, you can have water melon juice or banana. You can add ghee on navel at night. These tips will heal your constipation.

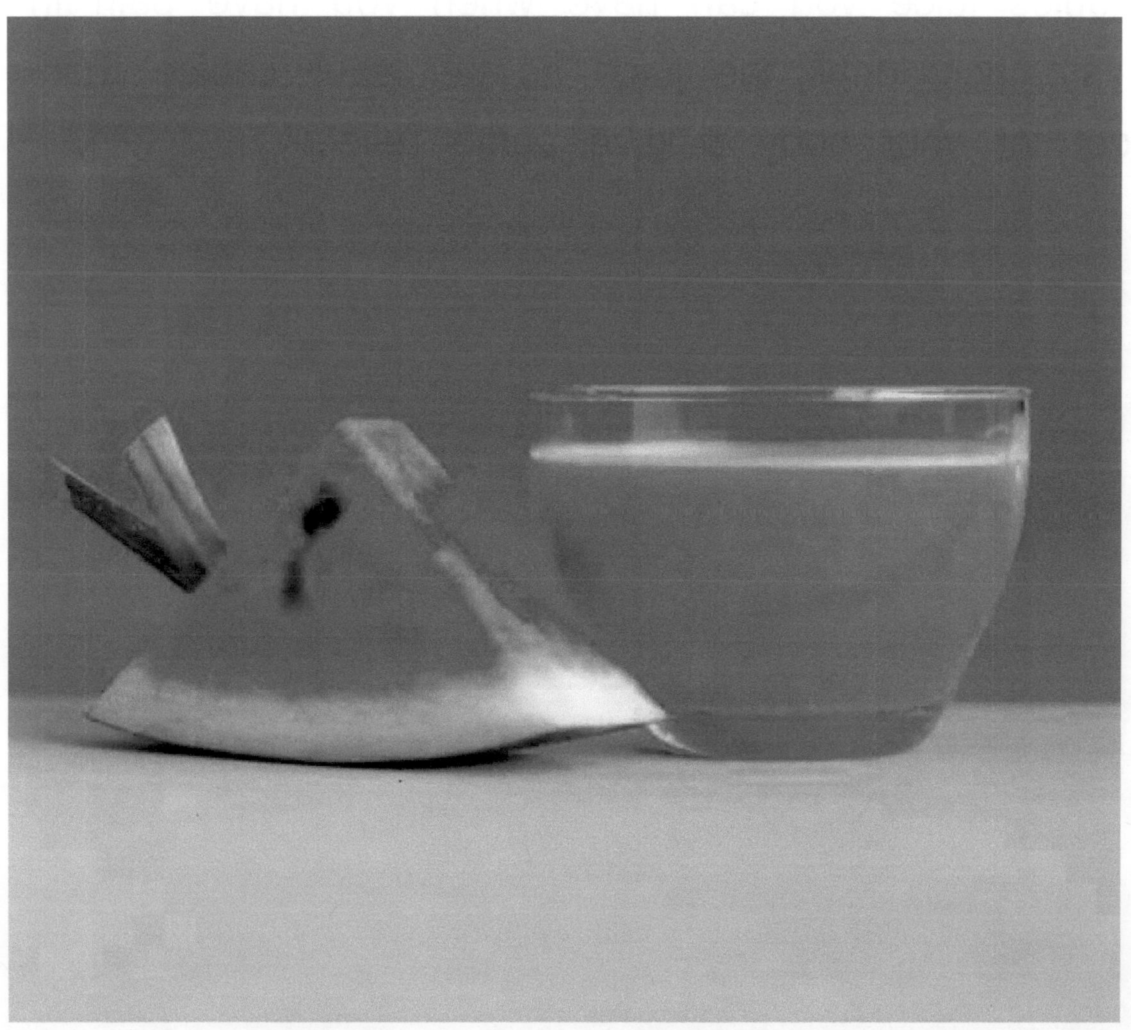

Stomach Pain:

First do light coconut oil massage on your stomach in circular motion (clock wise), you can try the juice listed & have juice which is best for your stomach.

1) Coconut juice 2) Spinach juice 3) Bitter Gourd juice (you can boil or grind) 4) Orange juice 5) Black grapes juice 5) Pear juice etc these are some fruits & vegetables juice you can have when you have pain in your stomach, drink the juice as per your choice that is cool for your body & give some relief.

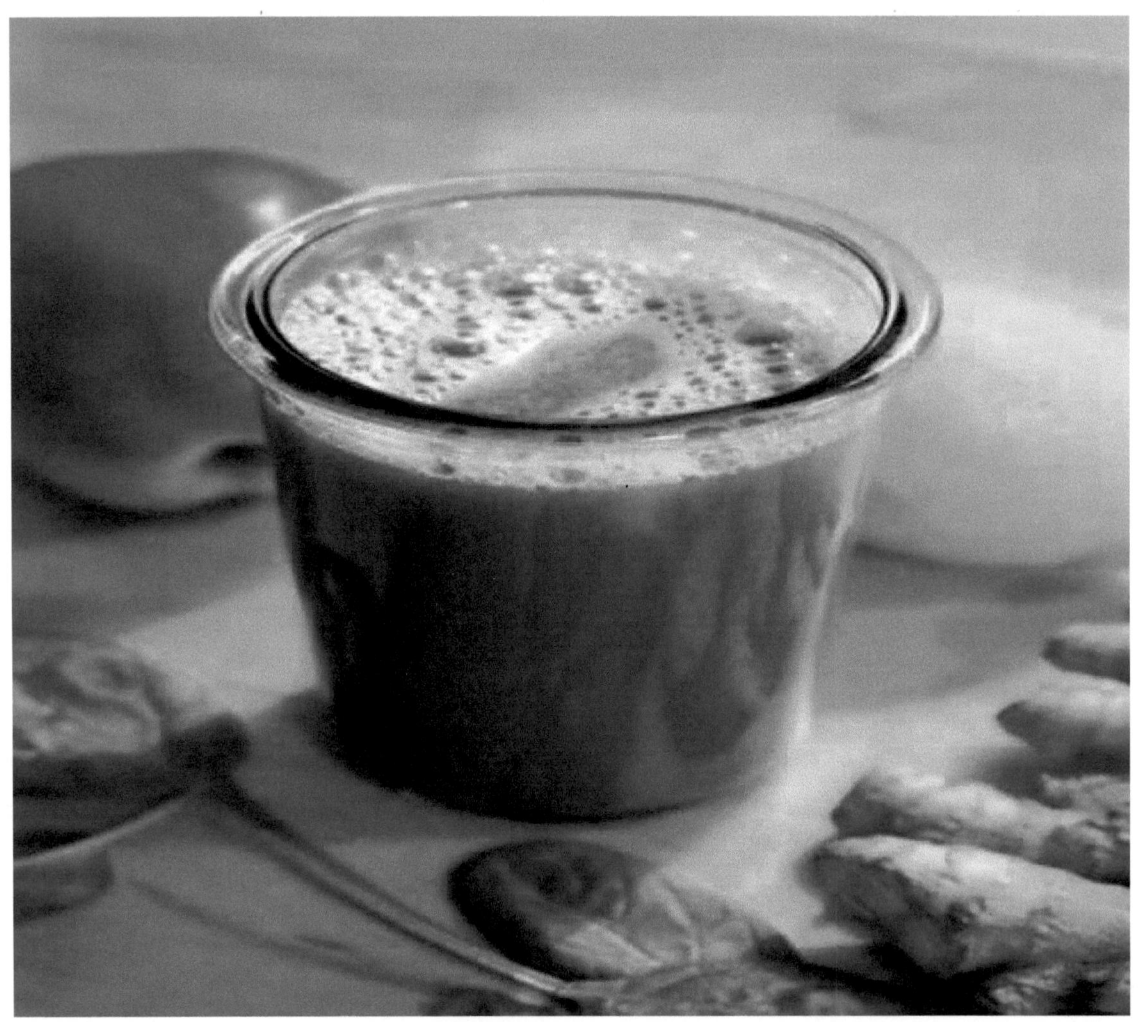

Periods: For over bleeding periods, you can have or make juice of North Indian rosewood or sheesham juice in the morning & evening, when it stops then no need to have. Make sure you should have plenty of water sip by sip during the day time. Vegetables like spinach, cucumber and in fruit like pomegranate that you can add to your diet.

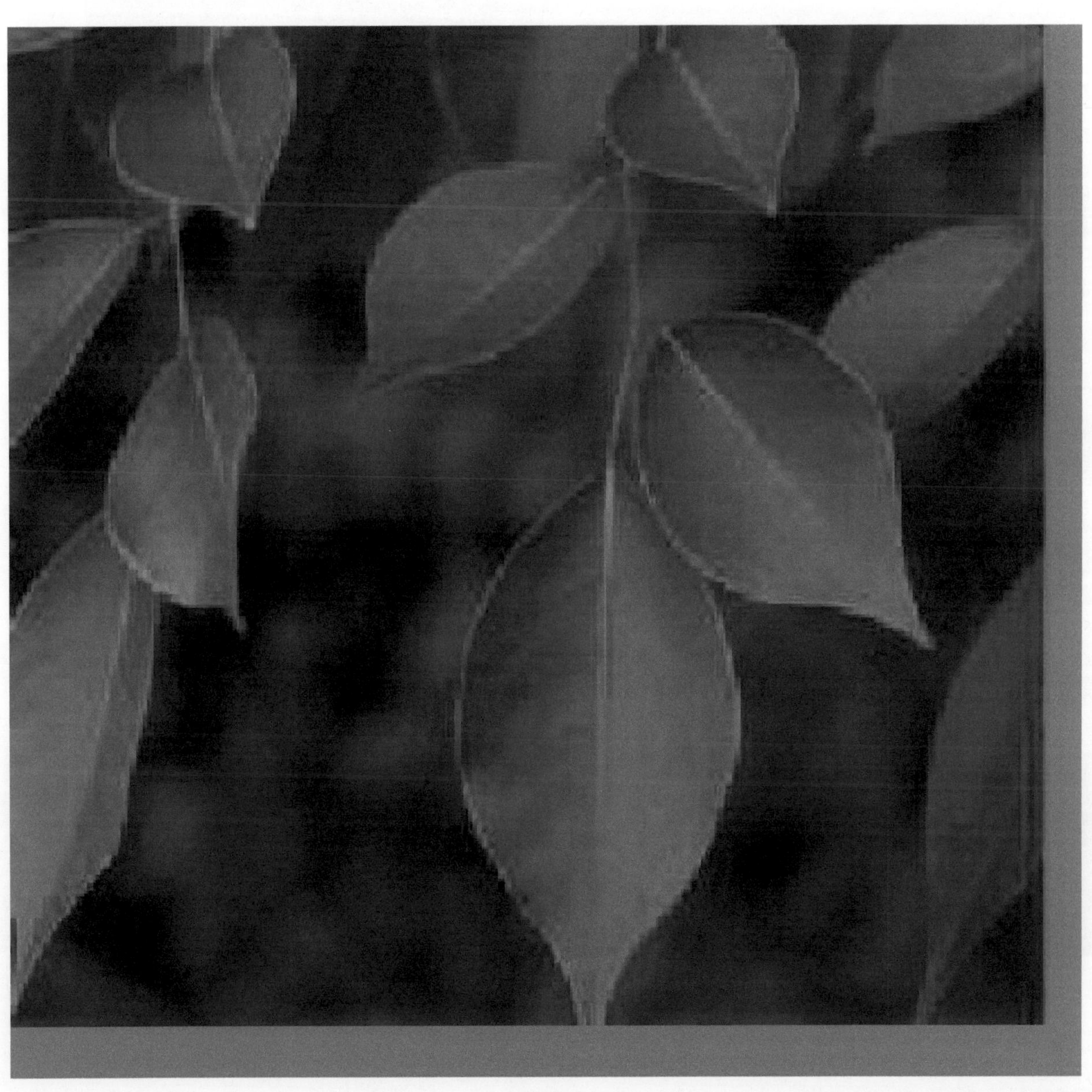

Acne: Drink Pineapple juice and also apply this juice on your acne area for 15 minutes and rinse off with rose water

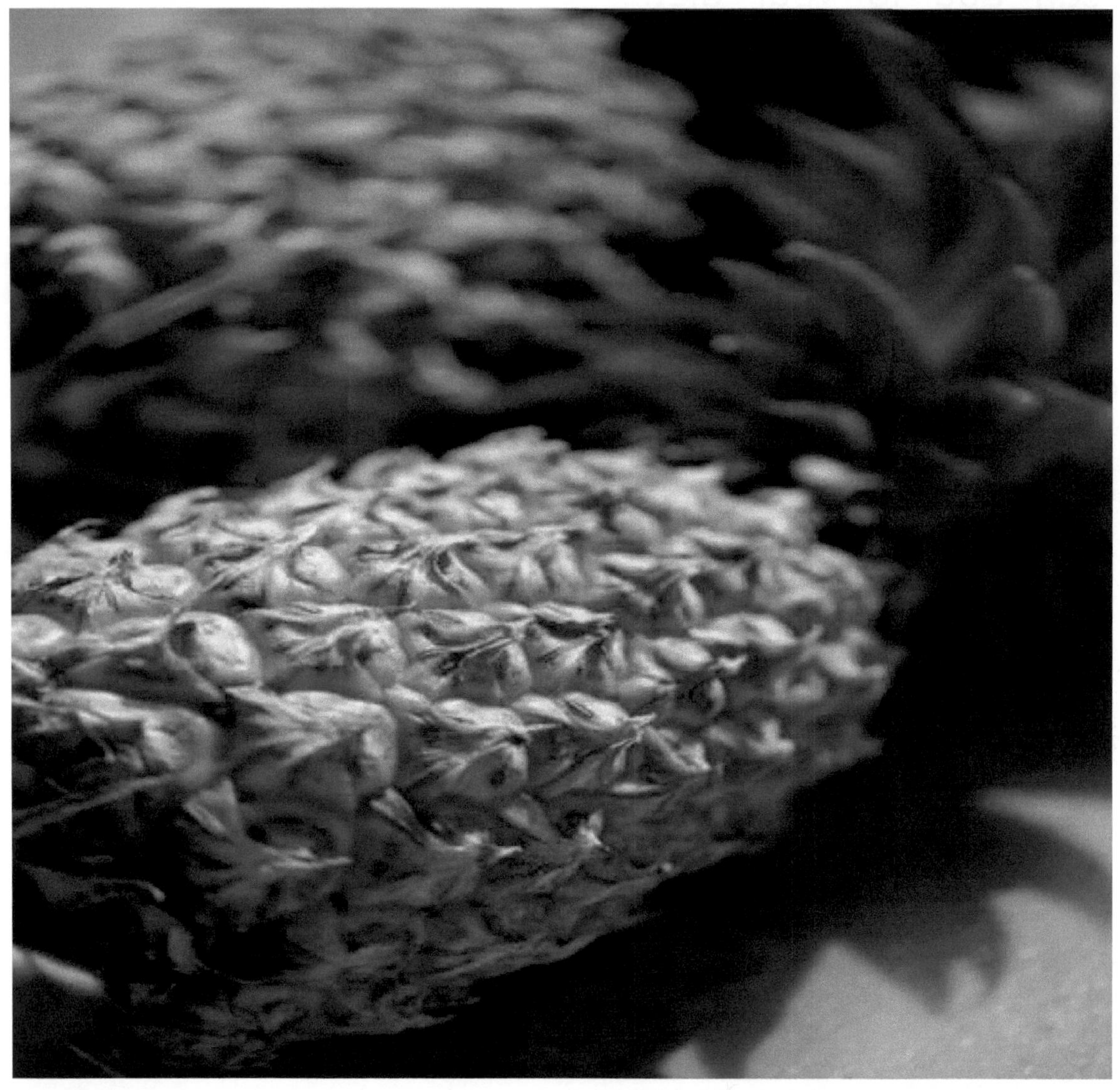

Diabetes: You can have bitter gourd and gooseberry juice together at equal quantity 2 times a day. You also have oats soup, pears and other common diet;

keep the diet less spicy & oil free. And do some Yoga; Kapalbathi & Manduka Aasans are very important to control sugar level.

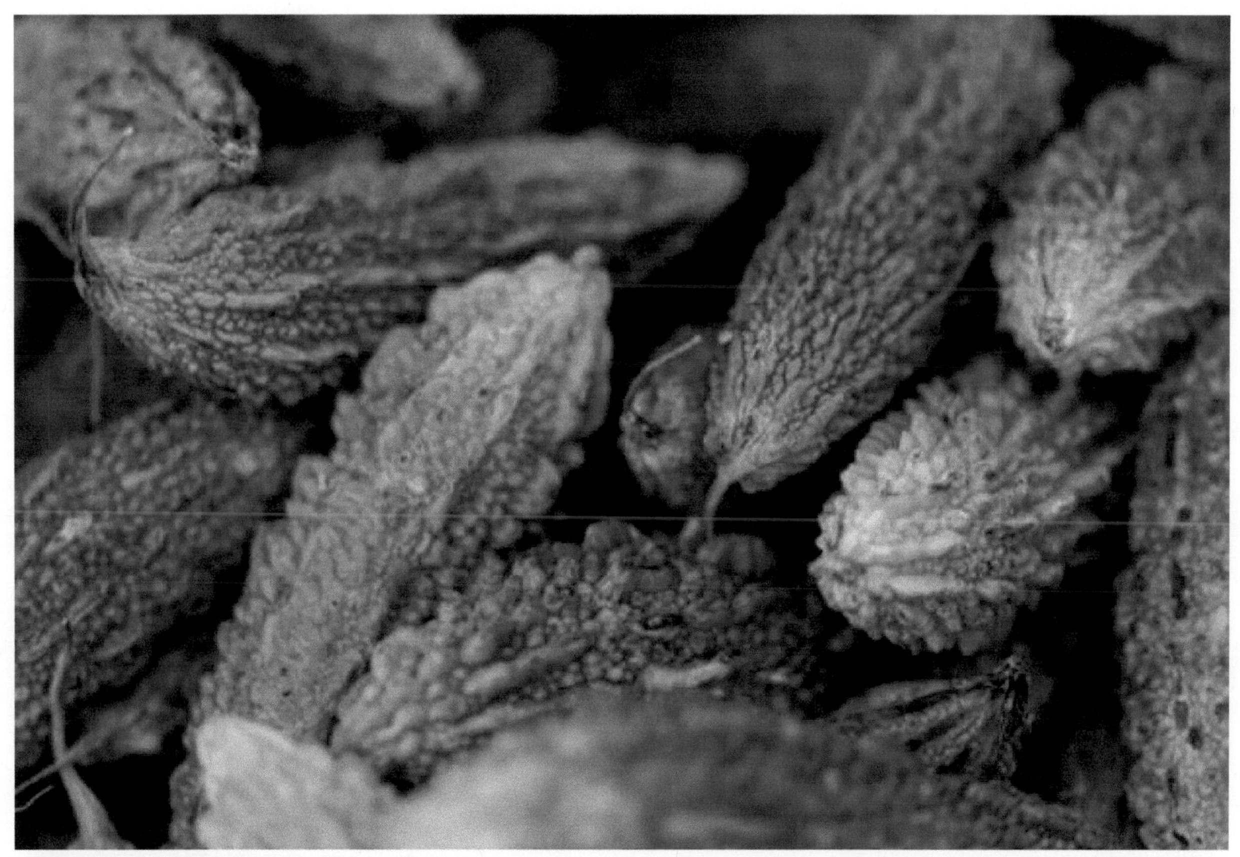

Eyes:

Eyes exercises will help you to improve your eyesight. You can try this exercise to improve, first roll your eyes to left, right, up & down, repeat 3 to 5 times.

Next keep your pointer finger in front of you to some distance then move your finger to right side but don't move your head right side only your eyes & hand coordination should be there, do the same process for the left side too.

You can also improve your eyesight when you connect with nature, breathe in fresh air and have fruits and vegetables that mother earth has given us.

You can try juice to improve your eyesight, drink orange juice in empty stomach & add 2 almond nuts on it.

You can have Spinach & carrot on your daily diet.

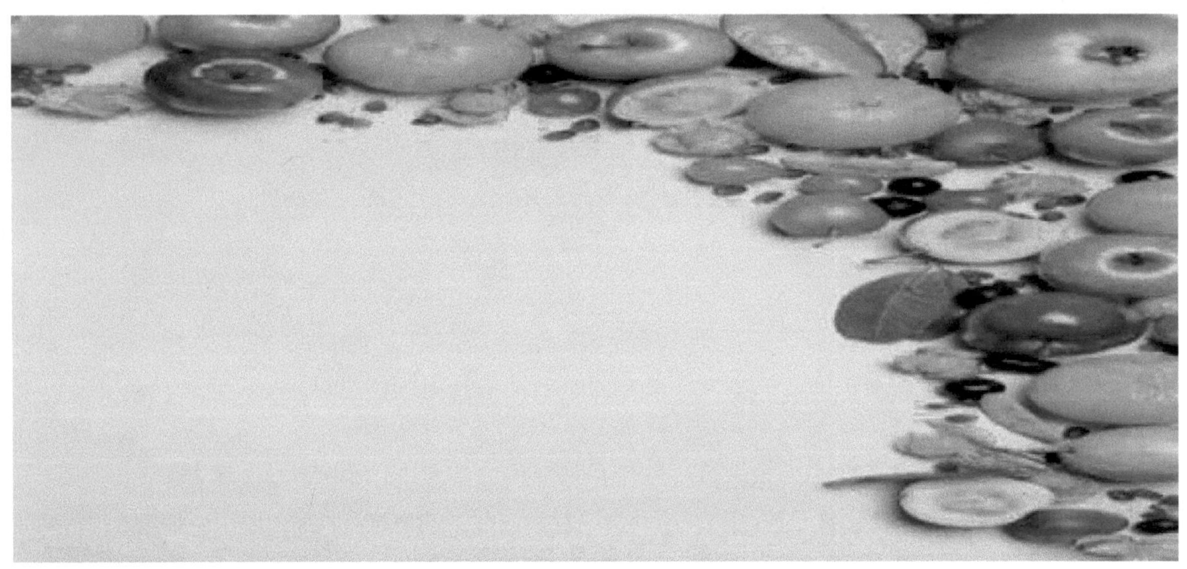

Skin: For any skin, Aloe Vera gel apply on your skin (face or whole body) and have Aloe Vera juice with fiber 1 or 2 table spoon at night before going to bed, after 1 hour of dinner.

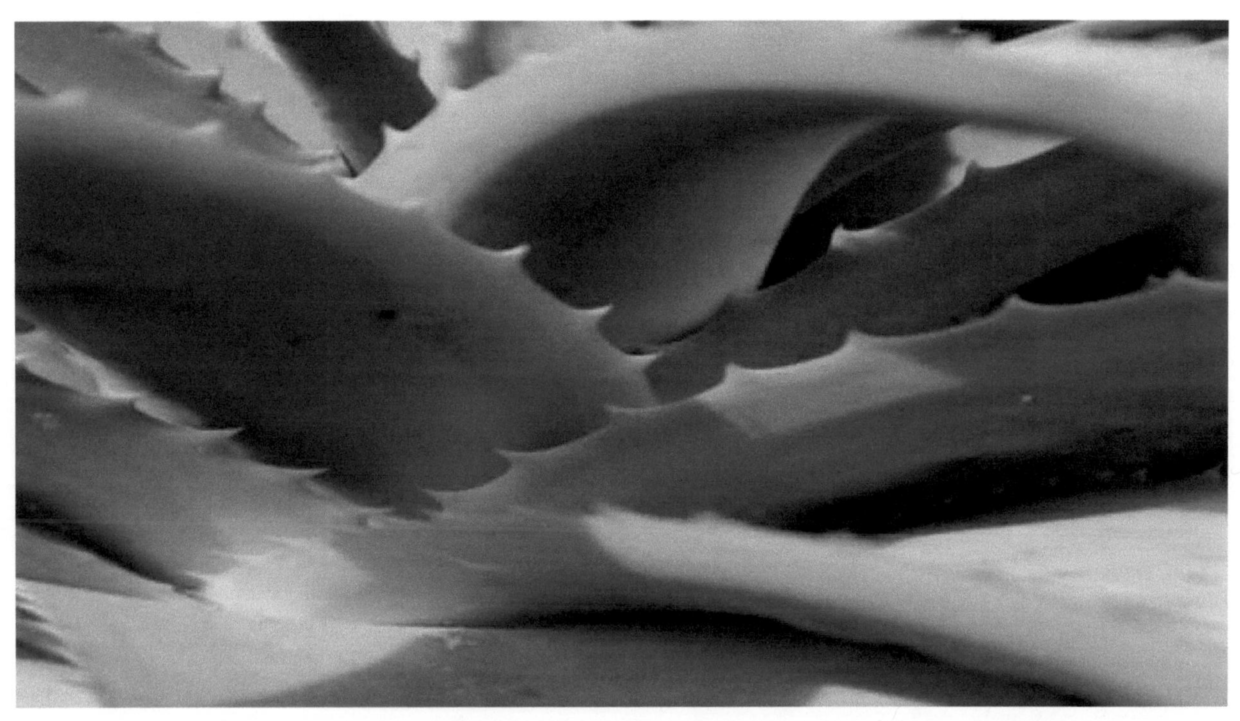

Tooth Pain: Grind Clove 10, cardamom 2, Black Pepper 5 to 8 seeds, Fenugreek seeds 1tsp and pinch of Pink or Sendha salt together make a powder & put a pinch of mixed powder on the area & wait for 20 seconds. For Tooth pain acupressure point for teeth will give great results.

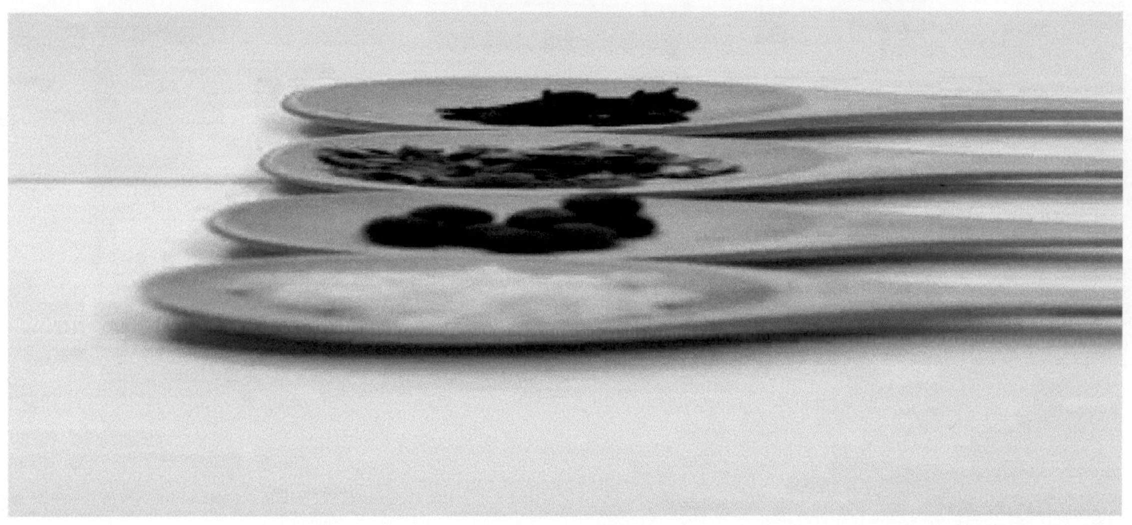

To cool your body: You can cool yourself by drinking fresh Spinach juice or Kale juice, and cucumber etc. At night apply Cow Ghee on navel, it cools your body or you can apply coconut oil on your stomach, do massage in circular motion (clockwise) in the morning will be of great help.

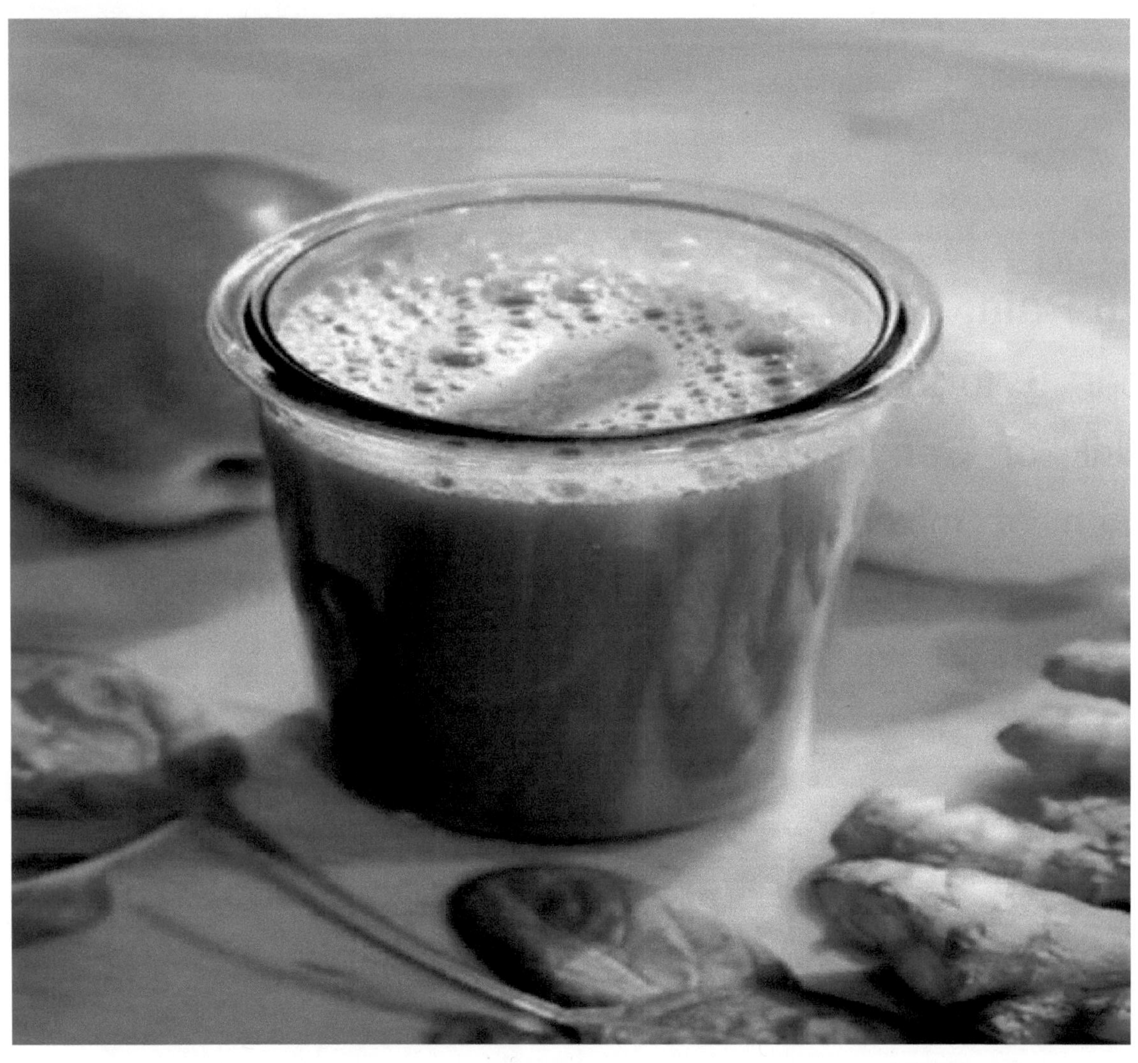

Weight loss: Don't sit in one place for longer time; add carom seeds to your diet. Add oil free food on your diet & don't keep your stomach empty for longer time, have sip of water instead. Add some routine exercises & yoga in your life.

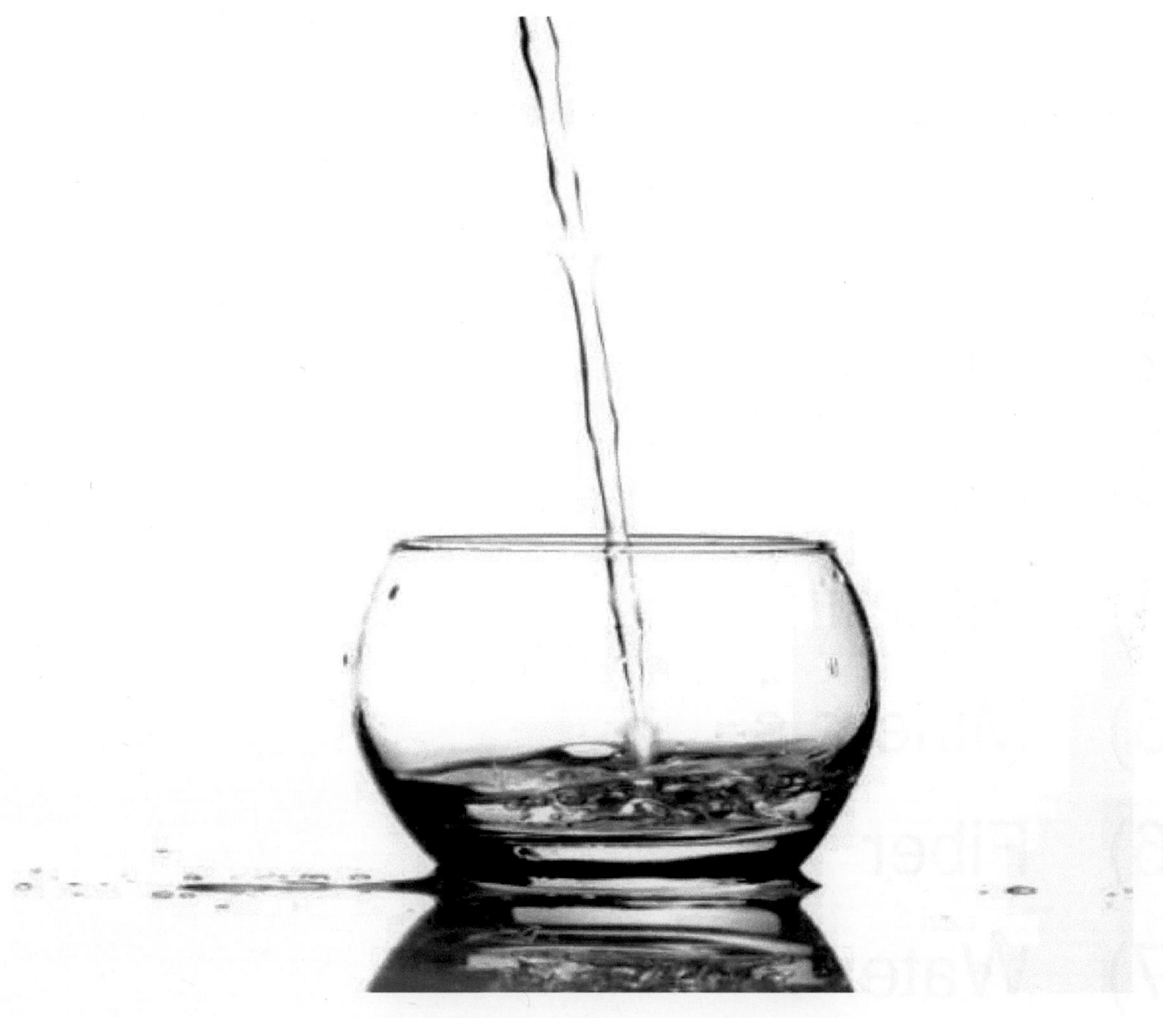

That's it......

Nutrients

Nutrients are substances found in our food that we consume. There are 7 nutrients that requires in our body on daily basis. These nutrients maintain our body.

1) Carbohydrates
2) Proteins
3) Fats
4) Vitamins
5) Minerals
6) Fiber
7) Water

Some best foods with high nutrients are listed below:

1) **Carbohydrates:** Milk, Beans, Popcorn, Potatoes, Spaghetti

2) **Proteins:** Include eggs, dairy products, fish and sea food, nuts: almonds, legumes, pumpkin seeds, peanuts, guava etc.

3) **Fats:** Nuts & Chocolates

4) **Vitamins:** It helps our body to function properly. **There are 13 Vitamins in our body. These Vitamins are divided into 2 types.**

Vitamin A, D, E & K are **fat soluble.**

Vitamin B & C are **water soluble.**

Vitamin A: Carrot, Broccoli, Sweet Potato, Kale, Turnip, Spinach, Tomato Mango, Water Melon, Apricot, Tangerine, Guava etc.

Vitamin B: Eggs, Leafy Greens, Legumes/pulses, Dairy Products, Seafood, plant seeds etc.

Vitamin B has different types of Vitamins.

B1 (Thiamin)
B2 (Riboflavin)
B3 (Niacin)
B5 (Pantothenic Acid)
B6 (Pyridoxine)
B7 (Biotin)
B9 (Folic acid)
B12 (Cyanocobalamin)

Vitamin C: Pineapples, Gooseberries, Strawberries, Oranges, Apples, Bananas, Guavas, Grape Fruit.

Vitamin D: For Vitamin D, you connect with nature; Sunlight & Eggs keeps our bones strong.

Vitamin E: Mango, Kiwi, Avocado etc,

Vitamin K: Most common food with high vitamin K such as blueberries, raspberries, plums, grapes, and figs are good for bones and in vegetables Kale, Broccoli, Spinach, Cabbage, & Lettuce.

5) **Minerals:** 7 major minerals include are Sodium, Potassium Chloride, Sulfur, Phosphorus, Calcium, and Magnesium.

You can find Minerals in food like cereals, nuts, fruits & vegetables, milk & dairy foods.

6) **Fiber:** You get good amount in berries of all kinds such as blueberries, raspberries, strawberries and blackberries like fruit, whole vegetables have a lot of fiber too.

7)Water: 70 percent of water is required for our body; that includes plain water & complete food we had throughout the day.

Drink loads of water that is sufficient for our system because water lubricates joints and helps bring calcium and other nutrients to your bones.

Other essential nutrients are Iron, Potassium, Calcium, Magnesium, Zinc, and Phosphorus.

Some regular food you need to add in your diet to get other essential nutrients like Iron, Potassium, Calcium, Magnesium, Zinc, and Phosphorus.

Calcium is important for bone health, muscles nervous system & circulatory system. Oats are high in calcium so you can opt for,

Almonds, Walnuts, Hazelnuts, Sesame seeds, Pumpkin & Sunflower seeds. Rich fruits like Apples, Figs, Oranges, and Blackberries.

Okay..........That's it for now.

I hope this book will be valuable to you & your family members. Thank you once again for choosing this book. Please take initiative to act & improve your health & of others and live a wonderful life.

One more thing...

If you really gained some knowledge from this book.

Please don't forget to give your valuable review on Amazon site about this book.

This will help the author to write more of such healthy tips books to improve the health of people.

Please share with others, may be this book will be of great help for them

I personally keep this book to follow & act, what about you?

Thank You!

Printed by Libri Plureos GmbH in Hamburg,
Germany